Introduction to Perfusion Quantification
using Arterial Spin Labeling

T0177535

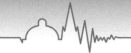

Oxford Neuroimaging Primers

Series Editors: Mark Jenkinson and Michael Chappell

Introduction to Neuroimaging Analysis
Mark Jenkinson
Michael Chappell

Introduction to Resting State fMRI Functional Connectivity
Janine Bijsterbosch
Stephen Smith
Christian Beckmann

**Introduction to Perfusion Quantification using
Arterial Spin Labeling**
Michael Chappell
Bradley MacIntosh
Thomas Okell

OXFORD NEUROIMAGING PRIMERS

Introduction to
Perfusion Quantification using Arterial Spin Labeling

MICHAEL CHAPPELL

BRADLEY MACINTOSH

THOMAS OKELL

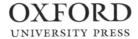

OXFORD
UNIVERSITY PRESS

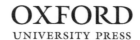

OXFORD
UNIVERSITY PRESS

Great Clarendon Street, Oxford, OX2 6DP,
United Kingdom

Oxford University Press is a department of the University of Oxford.
It furthers the University's objective of excellence in research, scholarship,
and education by publishing worldwide. Oxford is a registered trade mark of
Oxford University Press in the UK and in certain other countries

Published in the United States of America by Oxford University Press
198 Madison Avenue, New York, NY 10016, United States of America

British Library Cataloguing in Publication Data
Data available

Library of Congress Control Number: 2017949925

ISBN 978-0-19-879381-6

Printed in Great Britain by
Ashford Colour Press Ltd, Gosport, Hampshire

Preface to the Series

The Oxford Neuroimaging Primers are aimed to be readily accessible texts for new researchers or advanced undergraduates in neuroimaging who want to get a broad understanding of the ways in which neuroimaging data can be analyzed and interpreted. All primers in this series have been written so that they can be read as stand-alone books, although they have also been edited so that they "work together" and readers can read multiple primers in the series to build up a bigger picture of neuroimaging and be equipped to use multiple neuroimaging methods.

Understanding the principles of the analysis of neuroimaging data is crucial for all researchers in this field, not only because data analysis is a necessary part of any neuroimaging study, but also because it is required in order to understand how to plan, execute, and interpret experiments. Although MR operators, radiologists, and technicians are often available to help with data collection, running the scanner, and choosing good sequences and settings, when it comes to analysis, researchers are often on their own. Therefore, the Oxford Neuroimaging Primers seek to provide the necessary understanding of how to do analysis while at the same time trying to show how this knowledge relates to being able to perform good acquisitions, design good experiments, and correctly interpret the results.

The series has been produced by individuals (both authors and editors) who have developed neuroimaging analysis techniques, used these methods on real data, packaged them as software tools for others to use, taught courses on these methods, and supported people around the world who use the software they have produced. We hope that this means everyone involved has not only the experience to instruct, but also the empathy to support the reader. It has been our aim for these primers to not only lay out the core principles that apply in any given area of neuroimaging, but also to help the reader avoid common pitfalls and mistakes (many of which the authors themselves probably made first). We also hope that the series is also a good introduction to those with a more technical background, even if they have to forgo some of the mathematical details found in other more technical works. We make no pretense that these primers are the final word in any given area, and we are aware that the field of neuroimaging continues to develop and improve, but the fundamentals are likely to remain the same for many years to come. Certainly some of the advice you will find in these primers will never fail you—such as *always look at your data*.

Our intention with the series has always been to support it with practical examples, so that the reader can learn from working with data directly and will be equipped to use the knowledge they have gained in their own studies and on their own data. These examples, including datasets and instructions, can be found on the associated website (www.neuroimagingprimers. org), and directions to specific examples are placed throughout each primer. As the authors are also the developers of various software tools within the FMRIB Software Library (FSL), the examples in the primers mainly use tools from FSL. However, we intend these primers to be as general as possible and present material that is relevant for all readers, regardless of the software they use in practice. Such readers can still use the example data available through the primer website with any of the major neuroimaging analysis toolboxes. We encourage all readers to interact with these examples, since we strongly believe that a lot of the key learning is done when you actually use these tools in practice.

Mark Jenkinson
Michael Chappell
Oxford, January 2017

Preface

Arterial spin labeling (ASL) is an increasingly popular tool to study the brain. What sets it apart from other neuroimaging methods is the combination of quantitative measurements of a physiologically well-defined process, namely, perfusion, and a completely non-invasive acquisition methodology. Cerebral perfusion is a critical component of brain health, since it is the primary means of delivering nutrients to support brain function as well as of clearing waste products. Hence, it is a useful quantity to study in disease, where changes in perfusion can indicate regions of the brain that are pathological. Likewise, changes in perfusion can be indicative of greater demand for nutrients, such as might be required in response to an increase in neuronal activity.

While ASL has been in existence for over 15 years, for a variety of reasons, uptake and widespread usage of this perfusion neuroimaging tool have been slower than blood oxygenation level dependent (BOLD) techniques. This has been due partly to the apparently vast array of different ASL variants that have arisen as a result of the active development of improvements to the basic methodology. With the advent of a consensus by the ASL community on good practice and a recommendation on robust methods for ASL data collection, more and more researchers are now able to access and use ASL.

Despite the technological advances, ASL remains a technique with a low signal-to-noise ratio. This makes a wise choice of the appropriate analysis methods more important. While the ASL field has reached a consensus on acquisition, details on the choice of analysis methodology, especially in the context of neuroimaging studies, are still scattered throughout the literature. This was the context that led us to write this primer, with the aim of equipping someone new to the field of perfusion imaging and ASL with the knowledge not only to make good choices about ASL acquisition and analysis, but also to understand what choices they are making and why. To make this primer as helpful as possible, we illustrate the text throughout with examples of analysis applied to real data; you will find this data along with instructions on how to reproduce the analyses illustrated on the primer website: www.neuroimagingprimers.org.

This primer contains several different types of boxes in the text that are designed to help you navigate the material or find out more information for yourself. To get the most out of this primer, you might find the following descriptions of each type of box helpful.

Example Boxes These boxes illustrate the analysis methods discussed in the text on real ASL data. They also direct you to the Oxford Neuroimaging Primers website: www.neuroimagingprimers.org, where you will find the data used in each example along with instructions on how to perform the analysis for yourself. These examples are intended to be a useful way to prepare you

> **Example Box 1.1: A standar**
>
> The data acquired using our "stand
> volumes out of 61); this was acquir
> consensus paper, a label duration

for applying these methods to your own data, but you do not need to carry out these examples as you read through the primer.

Box 1.1: What is the differe

One way to distinguish between blc
Blood flow is strictly a measure of vc
Perfusion, being a measure of *delive*

Boxes These boxes contain more technical or advanced descriptions of some topics covered in this primer or information on related topics or methods. None of the material in the rest of the primer assumes that you have read these boxes, and they are not essential for understanding and applying any of the methods. If you are new to the field and are reading this primer for the first time, you may prefer to skip the material in these boxes and come back to them later.

SUMMARY

■ ASL works by creating magneti
  borne tracer.
■ ASL generates perfusion imag
  control conditions.

Summary Each chapter contains a box of summary points toward the end, which provide a very brief overview, emphasizing the most important topics discussed in each chapter. You may like to use these to check that you have understood the key points in each chapter.

FURTHER READING

■ Alsop, D. C., Detre, J. A., Go
  et al. (2015). Recommended i
  clinical applications: A consens
  Consortium for ASL in Dementi

Further reading Each chapter ends with a list of suggestions for further reading, including both articles and books. A brief summary of the contents of each suggestion is included, so that you can choose which references are most relevant to you. None of the material in this primer assumes that you have read any of the further reading material. Rather, these lists suggest a starting point for diving deeper into the existing literature. These lists are not intended to provide a full review of the relevant literature; should you go further into the field, you will find a wealth of other sources that are helpful or important for the specific research you are doing.

Like all areas of neuroimaging, ASL will continue to develop in the coming years, and new acquisition and analysis options will become available. Thus, this primer is not the last word in ASL perfusion imaging, but we hope that it will provide a comprehensive overview of the most commonly used methods for acquisition and analysis. We also hope that this will provide a good preparation for anyone delving deeper into the literature on ASL perfusion imaging.

Michael Chappell
Bradley MacIntosh
Thomas Okell

Acknowledgments

We are grateful to a host of people who have helped in the preparation of this primer. Particular thanks are due to Joseph Woods, Andrew Segerdahl, and Melvin Mezue, who provided a large proportion of the data we have used in the examples in this primer. We are very grateful to Mark Jenkinson, James Larkin, Manon Simard, and Andy Segerdahl for reading large portions of the primer and providing a wealth of helpful feedback.

We are also very grateful to a large number of people with whom we have worked over the years and who have provided inspiration, advice, and ideas that have ultimately helped our understanding of the topic of perfusion imaging and analysis, including Peter Jezzard, Manus, Donahue, Moss Zhao, Daniel Gallichan, Jingyi Xie, and Mark Woolrich. Honorable mentions are also due Adrian Groves, Daniel Bulte, David Crane, David Shin, David Thomas, Enrico De Vita, Esben Petersen, Federico von Samson-Himmelstjerna, Flora Kennedy McConnell, Illaria Boscolo Galazzo, Jesper Anderson, Marco Castellaro, Matthias Günther, Matthias van Osch, Michael Kelly, Nicholas Blockley, Samira Kazan, Stephen Payne, Thomas Liu, Wouter Teeuwisse, Xavier Golay, and Zahra Shirzadi.

Michael Chappell
Bradley MacIntosh
Thomas Okell

Contents

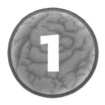

Introduction

Arterial spin labeling (ASL) magnetic resonance imaging (MRI) is unique in being a completely non-invasive method for imaging perfusion in the brain. As a perfusion imaging method, it is able to tell us about blood flow generally, but more specifically the delivery of blood to tissue, where blood has a role in transporting nutrients and removing waste. Like other perfusion imaging methods, ASL relies upon a blood-borne *tracer*, but, unlike other approaches (such as dynamic susceptibility contrast MRI or even positron emission tomography methods), it does not require the injection of a contrast agent. Instead, the ASL tracer is created by the MRI scanner itself. This makes it one of the most rapid and most participant-friendly ways to acquire perfusion images. Additionally, ASL not only creates perfusion-weighted images, but also provides quantitative measures of perfusion itself and not simply surrogate measures. This is potentially a great strength of ASL perfusion imaging, since quantitative measures should have the same meaning when collected on different days, on different scanners, and at different sites.

ASL relies upon a relatively simple modification to a standard MRI acquisition: before collection of the brain image, blood in the neck is converted into an MR tracer by the process of magnetic inversion of the hydrogen nuclei in water, commonly called *labeling*. In the simplest terms, the magnetic state of all of the water in a region of the neck is altered, which is useful because the water in the arterial blood is carried toward the brain in the bloodstream. After a delay period, this allows for the blood to travel from the place where it has been labeled, and this labeled blood-water arrives in the brain, where it accumulates within the tissue by crossing from the blood into cells and the spaces between the cells. The image acquired after the delay then contains information about the delivery of the tracer to the tissue. By comparing with a control image, where no labeling has been done, an image of perfusion can be obtained. Hence, the basic ASL experiment contains a pair of images: *label* and *control*. A typical acquisition collects multiple pairs of images to improve the signal-to-noise ratio (SNR). In some cases, extra information about hemodynamics is obtained by using a number of measurements with different delays post labeling: from such data, we can obtain information about the time required for blood to pass through parts of the vasculature.

The purpose of this primer is to provide an introduction to ASL, focusing on the methods needed to extract perfusion-weighted images from ASL data and quantify perfusion and other hemodynamic parameters, such as arterial transit time and arterial cerebral blood volume. This first chapter provides a brief overview of the simplest and most standard ASL acquisition and the steps for subsequent analysis. This process is illustrated using examples based on real ASL, and the discussion is linked to associated online example material where you can undertake the analysis for yourself. Subsequent chapters expand upon the basic material and provide more detail about common acquisition methods and the major analysis steps, with further illustrative examples. Later chapters provide information on more advanced analysis techniques, as well as how ASL-based perfusion information can be used in neuroimaging studies.

1.1 Measuring perfusion

What is perfusion and why are we interested in measuring it? Since you are reading this primer, you probably have some answers to these questions, but it is helpful to consider them at the outset. The definition of perfusion is apparently simple, but in practice people have slightly different interpretations, so we will state our working definition here. Perfusion is typically defined as the process of delivering nutrients, like oxygen and glucose, to the capillary bed. This inherently implies that only capillaries are responsible for perfusion, but in fact the different components of the vascular system, like arterioles and venules, play a role in perfusion; see Figure 1.1. Large blood vessels, like arteries or veins, are the necessary "pipes" that supply and drain blood from an organ, so enabling the flow of blood, and therefore, by acting as conduits for blood, they influence perfusion indirectly. In practice, the delivery of nutrients,

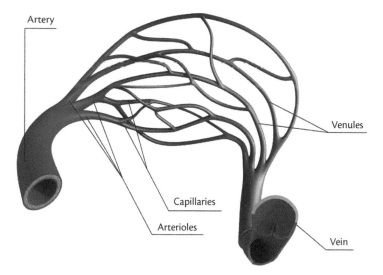

Figure 1.1: A conceptual illustration of the vasculature in body tissue. Blood passes from the main feeding artery into a branched structure of arterioles, which branch further to form a dense network of capillaries, where most of the exchange of nutrients and waste between blood and tissue occurs. The blood is drained from the tissue into venules and eventually veins.

> **Box 1.1: What is the difference between blood flow and perfusion?**
>
> One way to distinguish between blood flow and perfusion is to consider their respective units. Blood flow is strictly a measure of volume (of blood) per unit time, normally quoted in ml/min. Perfusion, being a measure of *delivery*, has units of volume of blood delivered to a volume (or mass) of tissue per unit time, typically quoted as ml (blood)/100g (tissue)/min. Thus, when it comes to perfusion, we need to know not only the volume of blood that is arriving, but also the volume into which it is distributed (and within which the transfer of nutrients happens).
>
> We can also define the blood volume, which measures the proportion of a given volume occupied by blood, typically quoted as the fractional volume of blood per volume (or mass) of tissue, e.g., ml (blood)/ml (tissue). This has similar-looking units to perfusion (being a volume of blood per volume of tissue), but omits time, and so relates to the static quantity of blood within the volume of tissue and not to the dynamic volume of blood arriving at the tissue.

such as oxygen, from the blood into cells can happen in every part of the vasculature and is not limited to the capillary bed, although this is where the majority of delivery occurs.

The physiology of perfusion can get complicated, especially in the context of pathology, but to all intents and purposes we view perfusion as the end product of the blood flow. In the case of the brain, we call this *cerebral blood flow*. The perfusion process naturally leads to consumption of oxygen and glucose consumption and to clearance of waste. At this point, you can go to the literature and notice that the terms perfusion and cerebral blood flow (or blood flow, when considering other organs) may be used interchangeably. At the risk of appearing pedantic, we should not be using these terms interchangeably, since they represent different things. A discussion on whether ASL measures perfusion or cerebral blood flow or both is outside the scope of this primer, although see Box 1.1 for more information on the differences, but generally it is understood that ASL can measure both of these hemodynamic phenomena.

With these definitions in mind, we can comfortably answer the question as to why one would want to measure perfusion. Succinctly, perfusion is a fundamental metric in physiology. Tissue cannot survive without adequate perfusion. It can also be an indicator of changes in metabolism in the tissue, reflecting changes in demand for nutrients that occur during neural activity or more gradually as a result of a disease process. Perfusion alterations can be dramatic, as in a stroke, or they can be more subtle and chronic, as observed in tumors, arteriovenous malformations, large artery stenosis, or neurodegenerative diseases such as vascular dementia. We might therefore suppose that perfusion can be an indicator of an upstream injury that prevents sufficient blood reaching a tissue and thereby leads to damage. ASL has been used to study all of these topics, as well as the spatial pattern of perfusion changes observed with age in the healthy population.

1.2 ASL acquisition

To keep things simple, we start by considering a "standard" ASL acquisition. We will follow the recommended acquisition from the ASL consensus paper (see Further Reading); a more detailed description of ASL acquisition will be given in Chapter 2. The ASL process is illustrated in Figure 1.2. In the simplest case, the way in which we get an image does not matter too much, and we will assume that we can acquire a full three-dimensional (3D) volume in a reasonable time using one of the popular ways of obtaining an image, such as echo planar imaging (EPI). As noted already, we need to acquire a pair of images, one with and one without labeling, and thus we need to define how this labeling will be achieved.

The consensus paper recommends pseudo-continuous labeling: typically referred to as pcASL. This defines a labeling plane in the neck, such that hydrogen nuclei within water molecules that pass through this plane experience a radiofrequency field that alters their magnetization (strictly speaking, it causes the magnetization to be inverted). This creates a tracer that is composed of labeled blood-water, which we will be able to detect in tissue based on the way it changes the images that we collect in the brain. This radiofrequency labeling continues for a pre-specified duration—the *label duration*—to create a well-defined volume of labeled blood-water. After labeling has occurred, there is a waiting time—the *post-label delay* (PLD)—to allow the labeled blood-water to pass through the vasculature, reach the brain tissue, and accumulate sufficiently that we can measure it. For example, the consensus paper recommends a label duration of 1.8 seconds and a PLD of 1.8 seconds for studies in healthy adults. Using our pcASL labeling, we can collect the label image, and, on subsequently acquiring another image without the radiofrequency labeling, we have a control image and thus a label–control pair, sometimes called a tag–control pair. This process will take around 9 seconds. The time for one image is around 4.5 seconds, including the 1.8 seconds of labeling, 1.8 seconds of the PLD, and a bit more time to acquire the brain image itself.

We are interested in the difference between label and control images, and this signal difference is typically around 1–2%, since the amount of labeled water that we can deliver by perfusion in the time of the ASL acquisition is small compared with the total volume of water in the tissue. This means that the SNR of the perfusion image will be inherently poor compared with the original images collected. You might ask why we do not label for even longer, thereby accumulating even more labeled water in the tissue and thus getting a bigger signal. The answer is that the label we have created is not permanent, and as soon as it has been created it starts to decay, disappearing over a period of a few seconds. The recommended acquisition parameters are a compromise between good delivery and limiting the effects of decay, something that we will consider further in Chapters 2 and 4.

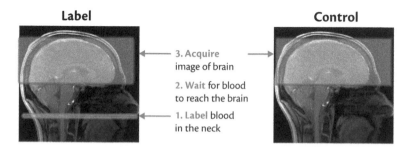

Label   **Control**

3. **Acquire** image of brain

2. **Wait** for blood to reach the brain

1. **Label** blood in the neck

Figure 1.2: The process of generating an ASL perfusion image relies on the acquisition of a pair of images: one with labeling of blood-water in the neck (label) and one without (control).

To get good quality perfusion images, we will need to repeat the acquisition a number of times and take an average of each intermediate perfusion pair. With 25 pairs, for instance, the total acquisition is 225 seconds (9 × 25). The consensus paper recommends that we also use *background suppression*, which means that we suppress the signal arising from the brain tissue itself, which has remained static between label and control images and is often called the *static tissue*. This approach aims to maximize our ability to find the difference between label and control images due to perfusion alone. Largely, it seeks to reduce artifacts arising from physiological sources (e.g., respiration) when we subtract pairs of images that would otherwise look like additional noise in the perfusion images—something we will consider further in Chapter 2.

If we want more than just a perfusion-weighted image (i.e., if we want the image intensity to reflect absolute perfusion in conventional units like ml/100g/min), then we need to know the "concentration" of our tracer. For this, we will need a separate image, in which we do not perform background suppression, for the purposes of quantification and calibration. Strictly speaking, the "concentration" of the label is given by the quantity called the *magnetization of arterial blood*, specifically that of the arterial blood that passed through the labeling plane. This magnetization is a property of the blood-water, and we can think of it as the available magnetization we have from which we can create the label. We cannot measure the magnetization of arterial blood directly, so we estimate it indirectly from elsewhere in the brain using the calibration image. For this calibration image, we will use exactly the same method to acquire the brain image, but we want the values in the image to be a measure of the magnetization of the brain tissues. This means that we want what is called a *proton-density-weighted image*, since this depends only on the magnetization of the hydrogen nuclei in water and not other properties of the tissue. This is normally achieved by using a long repetition time (TR) and a short echo time (TE). The long TR means there is more time between acquiring one image and the next, reducing the influence of the time-dependent T_1 relaxation process: a TR of more than 5 seconds is generally regarded as long enough. The short TE means that other sources of MR image contrast, namely, relaxation associated with T_2 and/or T_2^* effects, are minimized. An example of data collected using the consensus paper recommendations is shown in Example Box 1.1.

Example Box 1.1: A standard ASL dataset

The data acquired using our "standard" ASL sequence is shown in Figure 1.3 (only the first 24 volumes out of 61); this was acquired using pcASL labeling and 2D EPI imaging. Following the consensus paper, a label duration of 1.8 seconds with a PLD of 1.8 seconds was used. As 2D imaging was used to collect a full 3D volume, the PLD corresponds to the most inferior slice; for each subsequent slice, the PLD was increased by 45.2 ms (see Chapter 2). The imaging data has a matrix size of 64 × 64, with 24 slices, with voxel size of 3.4 mm × 3.4 mm × 5 mm. The repetition time (TR) was 4.8 seconds, and the data was acquired with a calibration image first, followed by label–control pairs in which background suppression had been applied.

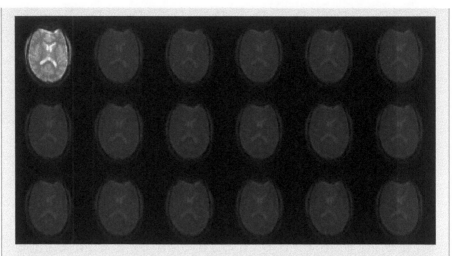

Figure 1.3: A single 2D slice within an ASL series. The first image is for calibration, and the following images are the individual volumes from the label–control pairs with background suppression applied. Only the first 24 images are shown.

Notice that the first image is much brighter than the rest; this is the calibration image. The rest are the individual volumes from the label–control pairs with background suppression applied, which has worked to remove most (but not all) of the tissue signal that can be seen in the calibration image. It happens that in this dataset the first of the ASL pairs (the second volume in the data overall) is a label image, followed by a control image—but this would be almost impossible to spot from the raw data. It is conventional to collect a label image before a control image, although there is no particular reason to do so.

1.3 ASL analysis

The generation of a *perfusion-weighted* image from ASL data is relatively simple, requiring the pairwise subtraction of label and control images to leave the contribution of labeled blood-water delivered by the vasculature. Since the magnitude of the signal directly relates to the delivery of blood, the image created is itself perfusion-weighted. The most prominent perfusion feature is the difference between gray and white matter: contrasting regions with high and low perfusion. To go beyond the perfusion-weighted image, and generate quantitative voxelwise measures of perfusion with values in the typical units of ml/100 g/min, we need an analysis scheme that should look like the following:

- subtraction
- kinetic modeling
- calibration

We will now briefly explain these concepts as applied to the basic ASL acquisition outlined already—a more complete and detailed description of each stage follows in Chapters 3–5.

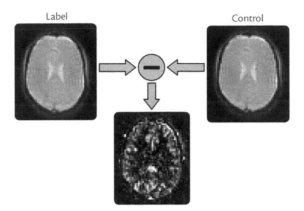

Label   Control

Figure 1.4: Subtraction of a label–control pair of images results in an image with perfusion weighting.

1.3.1 Subtraction

Central to ASL analysis is the subtraction of label and control images. We have established that both label and control images will contain some signal from brain tissue—which we called the static tissue signal—even if background suppression has been used to reduce this contribution. Subtraction of the label–control pair reveals the contribution from labeled blood-water as illustrated in Figure 1.4 (something that can be written quite simply mathematically, as we show in Box 1.2). This image is often referred to as the *difference image* and is perfusion-weighted, which means that it reflects the perfusion in each voxel, but the intensity value in each voxel does not alone provide an absolute measure of perfusion. As is typical of ASL data, a single difference image is quite noisy, and multiple images are acquired and averaged, something that we explore further in Example Box 1.2.

Box 1.2: **Label-control subtraction**

We can write the content of the label and control images (in each voxel) mathematically as

$$S_{label} = S_{static} - S_{blood}$$

$$S_{control} = S_{static} + S_{blood}$$

Notice that both images actually contain a contribution from the blood, but for the label image we have inverted the magnetization of the blood water, and thus it provides a negative contribution. Subtraction of these two images thus produces an image only related to the blood signal:

$$\Delta S = S_{control} - S_{label} = 2S_{blood}$$

Example Box 1.2: A perfusion-weighted image

Taking the "standard" data we examined in Example Box 1.1, ignoring the calibration image, and doing a pairwise subtraction of the remaining label–control pairs, i.e., volume 3 (first control image) minus volume 2 (first label image), volume 5 minus volume 4, etc., we arrive at the difference images in Figure 1.5. Notice how noisy each difference image is, but there is a noticeable pattern there that looks like a perfusion image should: namely, high intensity around the outer regions of the brain where the cortex is and lower intensity in areas dominated by white matter. Taking the mean over all the difference images gives the perfusion-weighted image, as shown in Figure 1.6. At this point, the intensities are still on the same scale as the data coming out of the scanner, which is arbitrary and depends on many MRI factors that do not pertain to absolute perfusion (e.g., gain settings of the MRI radiofrequency signal amplifiers). Notice how much smaller the magnitude of the perfusion-weighted image is than the raw data, shown alongside in Figure 1.6—in fact, the intensities in the perfusion-weighted image are of the order of 1% of those in the calibration image.

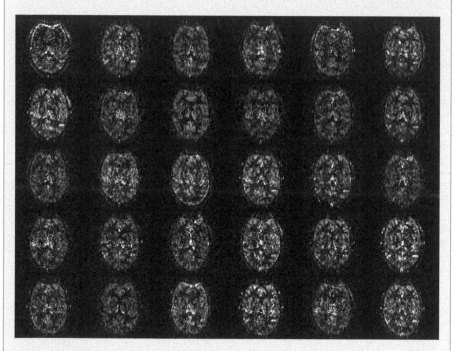

Figure 1.5: Difference images arising from subtraction of adjacent pairs of label and control images, showing the subtraction results from all 30 pairs.

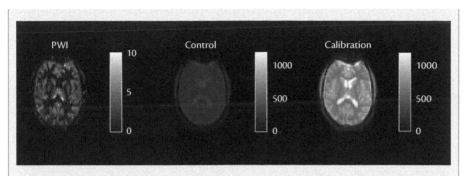

Figure 1.6: Left: Perfusion-weighted image (PWI)—the mean over all the label–control difference images (which are shown in Figure 1.5). Center: A single ASL volume with background suppression (a label image). Right: The calibration image. Note the differences in intensity scales on each of these images.

1.3.2 Kinetic modeling

The voxel intensity in an ASL difference image is directly related to the labeled blood-water. More accurately, it relates to the amount of labeled blood-water that has accumulated in the voxel in the time between the creation of the label and the collection of a brain image. This means that it is a measure of delivery and thus perfusion, rather than blood volume or blood flow rate. To be able to say how much labeled blood has been delivered, and thus what the perfusion is, it is necessary to describe the delivery process, as well as what happens to the labeled blood once it has been delivered. This is achieved by means of a kinetic model.

At its very simplest, the kinetic model for labeled blood-water in an ASL study needs to account for the delivery of a finite duration (the label duration) of labeled blood-water into the voxel where it accumulates. At the same time as it is being delivered, the label is also decaying away. The tracer decays at a rate defined by the T_1 time constant, which is of the order of a second in the brain at typical MRI field strengths. The ASL signal that we detect is therefore subject to the competing effects of how much label has arrived at a voxel relative to how much longer that tracer signal will last. In practice, the process that creates the label is imperfect, and it is necessary to account for how effective labeling has been; this can be expressed in terms of an efficiency, the *inversion efficiency*, since we can define what perfect labeling is and thus how far short we are.

The difference in magnitude between label and control images, the difference signal, thus depends upon the rate of delivery (perfusion), blood equilibrium magnetization, label duration, and T_1. The kinetic model allows the relationship between the signal and perfusion to be expressed as an equation, and this can be rearranged to give an equation that takes signal magnitude and returns perfusion. In practice, kinetic models can be used with varying degrees of sophistication, accounting for a range of other effects that might change the signal we measure, unrelated to perfusion, which is something we will consider further in Chapter 4.

1.3.3 Calibration

The ASL calculation relies on knowledge of the tracer concentration (strictly speaking, the quantity called the equilibrium magnetization of arterial blood), which will vary between individuals, and other MRI-related factors (e.g., the main magnetic field strength). As we have already noted, the simplest approach for estimating this parameter is by the acquisition of a separate proton-density-weighted image. This can be converted to a measure of arterial magnetization by accounting for the relative density of hydrogen nuclei in tissue and blood (the partition coefficient), something that we consider further in Chapter 5.

The process of subtraction, kinetic modeling, and calibration can, at least for the acquisition type we have considered in this chapter, be combined into a single formula that can be used for quantification as discussed in Box 1.3. Example Box 1.3 shows what happens when we apply kinetic modeling and calibration to ASL data.

Box 1.3: A simple equation for calculating perfusion

For the basic ASL technique described in this chapter, a simple kinetic model can be derived and converted to give the expression

$$CBF = \frac{6000\lambda(S_{control} - S_{label})e^{PLD/T_1}}{2\alpha T_1 S_{PD}(1 - e^{-\tau/T_1})}$$

Notice that this includes the label–control subtraction ($S_{control} - S_{label}$) as well as division by the magnitude of the proton-density-weighted image, S_{PD}. For our "standard" sequence, the post-labeling delay (PLD) is given by the sequence design as 1.8 s and the label duration τ is also 1.8 s. A standard value of T_1 for arterial blood is often used, taken from the literature to be 1.65 s at 3 T, as well as a standard value of the pcASL labeling efficiency α of 0.85 and a single whole brain partition coefficient value λ of 0.9 that accounts for the difference in proton (water) density between blood and brain tissue. The factor of 6000 that is included in the expression converts the final value into the standard ml/100g/min units.

Example Box 1.3: An image of absolute perfusion

To convert the perfusion-weighted image from Example Box 1.2 into a measure of absolute perfusion, we need the calibration data: the first volume in our dataset as shown in Figure 1.3. We can then apply the kinetic model to give the final absolute perfusion image as shown in Figure 1.7. This is what a typical perfusion image looks like; notice that there are some very high-intensity values around the edges of the brain that are artifacts of the division of the perfusion-weighted image by the calibration image in voxels at the edge of the brain that are only partially tissue. This is something we will discuss further in Chapter 5.

In fact, we can do a bit better than the result in Figure 1.7 by applying motion correction, using adaptive spatial smoothing and taking a different approach to calibration, all of which are discussed in later chapters. For the time being, an example of what you might be aiming for after reading the rest of this primer is shown in Figure 1.8.

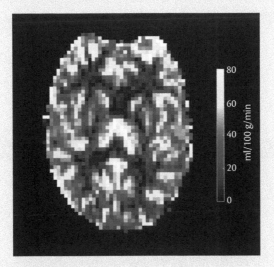

Figure 1.7: A single slice from the calculated absolute perfusion image in units of ml/100 g/min.

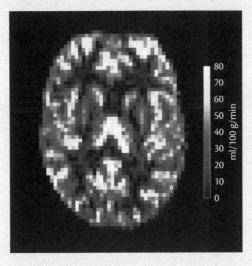

Figure 1.8: A single slice from the calculated absolute perfusion image (ml/100 g/min) when additional correction and processing has been applied.

On the primer website, you will find the dataset used in the examples in this chapter and instructions on how to compute the images shown, illustrating the complete process to obtain a quantified perfusion image from a standard ASL dataset.

SUMMARY

- ASL works by creating magnetically labeled blood-water in arteries in the neck as a blood-borne tracer.
- ASL generates perfusion images using pairs of images, alternating between label and control conditions.
- A perfusion-weighted image is obtained by subtraction of the label–control pair. Typically, an average is taken over multiple acquisitions to reduce noise.
- Absolute perfusion can be obtained by using a kinetic model together with the additional acquisition of a calibration image that gives a measure of the magnetization of arterial blood.

FURTHER READING

- Alsop, D. C., Detre, J. A., Golay, X., Günther, M., Hendrikse, J., Hernandez-Garcia, L., et al. (2015). Recommended implementation of arterial spin-labeled perfusion MRI for clinical applications: A consensus of the ISMRM Perfusion Study Group and the European Consortium for ASL in Dementia. *Magnetic Resonance in Medicine*, 73(1), 102–116.
  - *This paper, commonly called the "white paper," is now the main reference for anyone trying to do ASL. It was aimed primarily at making ASL more accessible and widely used, particularly for clinical applications, and thus recommends a simple, robust, and widely tested combination of acquisition and analysis options that we have discussed in this chapter. It goes on to discuss some further modifications and improvements that can be made to the basic ASL methodology. These enhancements may be particularly relevant for neuroimaging studies, where the questions to be answered differ from those in clinical applications.*
- Buxton, R. (2009). *Introduction to Functional Magnetic Resonance Imaging: Principles and Techniques* (2nd ed.). Cambridge University Press.
  - *This provides a useful and more detailed introduction both to MR physics and to neural physiology, along with an overview of the principles of both ASL and BOLD fMRI.*

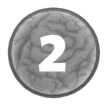

ASL Acquisition Principles

We have already described the basic ASL "experiment": label, wait, and then image; followed by another, control, image without labeling. In practice, there are a number of ways of achieving the label and control (which has to be carefully matched to the labeling process) and a variety of different ways of acquiring the associated brain images. There are also additional options that can be used to suppress artifacts or in attempts to improve image quality. This chapter seeks to provide an overview of the main concepts needed to choose a suitable ASL acquisition and extract the information needed for subsequent analysis. You might find that you only have certain options available to you on the scanner you are using, depending upon who has provided your ASL sequence. At the very least, this chapter should help you know what different terms mean and what it is you need to know about the ASL sequence you are using. Since ASL is very modular in nature (different ASL labeling schemes can be combined with different waiting approaches and readout methods), we will consider each part in turn.

2.1 Labeling

As we saw in Chapter 1, it is the process of labeling blood-water that uniquely allows ASL to measure perfusion using an endogenous tracer. To create a label, we have to manipulate the magnetic properties of the hydrogen nuclei in the water. These hydrogen nuclei are often called "spins" by MR physicists and this is why we talk about arterial *spin* labeling. We have already seen that labeling occurs in the neck using radiofrequency fields, which subject the hydrogen nuclei to a process called inversion. All the hydrogen nuclei in the body have a magnetization, and this quantity has both a magnitude and direction. When placed in a strong magnetic field (e.g., within an MRI scanner), these spins tend to align their direction with the applied field. Using radiofrequency fields, we can "tip" some spins into the opposite direction—inversion— and thereby create a label. In practice, the details are slightly more complex than this, and if you are interested you should consult the Primer Appendix: A Short Introduction to Magnetic Resonance Imaging Physics for Neuroimaging.

The literature on ASL can be quite confusing when you first come across it: there are a wide variety of ASL labeling schemes and variations on each of these, with a baffling array of associated acronyms (see Box 2.7 for some guidance). The ASL consensus paper produced by the ISMRM Perfusion Study Group and the European Consortium for ASL in Dementia (see Further reading) produced some clear guidelines on a simple and robust implementation of ASL, which should give good quality data in a wide variety of scenarios. The recommended labeling scheme is pseudo-continuous ASL (pcASL), which is now becoming widely adopted. However, there may be sites where pcASL is not available, or there may be technical reasons why pcASL cannot be used. For example, at high field strengths (7 T and above), the power absorbed by biological tissues in the pcASL labeling scheme may become prohibitive. Therefore, in this section, we briefly describe the main methods by which the labeling process can be performed, along with their main advantages and disadvantages. But first, we will consider some desirable characteristics for our labeling scheme that may help inform us about how to choose between possible options.

2.1.1 What do you want from a labeling scheme?

As we discussed in Chapter 1, the main aim of the labeling process is to invert, or label, the magnetization of arterial blood-water flowing into the brain, generating a signal change that we can detect, and from which we can estimate the perfusion. There are a number of characteristics that we would want from an ideal labeling scheme:

- **Efficient labeling**: To maximize the signal difference between label and control images, we want the magnetization of the arterial blood-water to be perfectly inverted during the labeling process. However, in practice, perfect inversion is difficult to achieve. The inversion efficiency α quantifies this effect, with $\alpha = 1$ corresponding to perfect inversion and $\alpha = 0$ to no inversion. Knowledge of α is important for accurate quantification of perfusion, as we shall see in Chapter 4.

- **Long label duration**: The longer the duration of the labeled bolus, the more labeled blood-water will accumulate in the tissue, leading to a larger ASL signal. This is somewhat counteracted by T_1 decay of the labeled blood-water, but label durations in the range 1.8–4 s are thought to be optimal for maximizing SNR.

- **Well-defined label duration**: The duration of the bolus of labeled blood is an important factor in the ASL kinetic model and thus the accuracy by which we can estimate perfusion, something we will consider further in Chapter 4. Methods that produce a bolus with a clearly specified label duration are therefore desirable.

- **Perfectly balanced control**: While inversion efficiency during labeling is important, it is also crucial that the control images are acquired in such a way that the blood signal is not affected (i.e., $\alpha = 0$) and that the static tissue signal is identical in both label and control conditions. Even fairly subtle effects, such as minor perturbations to the water signal resulting from the labeling, can be significant relative to the small perfusion signal we wish to measure.

- **Consistent labeling efficiency**: In order for perfusion to be accurately quantified, the labeling efficiency should be consistent across a reasonable physiological range. For example, we would not want it to change significantly when the velocity of blood in the feeding arteries changes, which may occur in disease or when certain drugs are administered.

- ■ **Insensitivity to magnetic field inhomogeneity**: Inhomogeneity, or unevenness, in the main magnetic field of the scanner, and in the radiofrequency fields, becomes more problematic at higher field strengths. Our ideal labeling scheme will be insensitive to variations in these fields.

- ■ **Minimal power deposition**: At high field strengths, particularly 7 T and higher, the amount of power deposited (absorbed by the tissues) by radiofrequency fields must be carefully controlled to avoid excessive heating. In these cases, labeling schemes with minimal power deposition are desirable.

2.1.2 Continuous ASL (cASL)

The original implementation of ASL used a continuous labeling scheme. This involves the use of a continuous radiofrequency field that is applied in the presence of a magnetic field gradient. When the parameters of the radiofrequency fields and gradients are chosen correctly, this results in the creation of a labeling plane: any magnetization flowing through this labeling plane is gradually rotated (or "tipped") in such a way that upon reaching the other side of this plane, the magnetization is pointing in the opposite direction (Figure 2.1). This process is technically known as flow-driven adiabatic inversion.

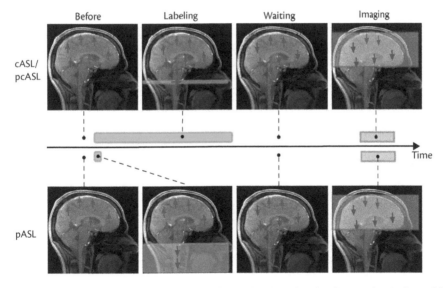

Figure 2.1: The process of magnetic inversion with cASL/pcASL and pASL. The time line in the middle indicates the timing of the different phases of the ASL labeling process. The timing and approximate duration of the applications of different radiofrequency fields are shown, including those relating to labeling (blue) and imaging (orange). Prior to labeling, all the blood-water magnetization (red arrows) is aligned with the main magnetic field. With cASL/pcASL, during the labeling period, any blood flowing through the defined labeling plane (blue line) is rotated so that it points in the opposite direction to the main magnetic field. With pASL, a single brief labeling pulse inverts all the blood magnetization within some spatial region (blue box). In both cases, inverted blood is then allowed to flow into the brain before imaging is performed (orange box).

In this manner, all blood flowing through the labeling plane while the radiofrequency fields and gradients are switched on is inverted. This creates a well-defined bolus of labeled blood-water with a label duration defined by how long the field was applied for.

Advantages of cASL:

■ Very efficient labeling.

■ Well-defined label duration.

■ Long label durations are achievable.

Disadvantages of cASL:

■ Cannot generally be performed on standard clinical scanners, since long continuous radiofrequency "pulses" are difficult to achieve without specialist equipment.

■ An effective control is difficult to achieve with this method, particularly for multi-slice experiments, since magnetization transfer effects (in which the water signal is slightly reduced owing to interactions with other large molecules that are also affected by the labeling process) tend to be significant.

■ Labeling efficiency depends somewhat on blood flow velocity.

2.1.3 Pulsed ASL (pASL)

In pulsed ASL, a single, relatively short (~10 ms), radiofrequency pulse is used to invert the magnetization over a specific region of space, encompassing the brain-feeding arteries, see Figure 2.1. Unlike cASL, therefore, the labeling is nearly instantaneous. In this case, since a spatial region is specified for labeling, the label duration is not known, since it will depend on the velocity of blood in the arteries. Achieving a longer label duration requires labeling a larger region of space. However, this can lead to a reduction in inversion efficiency for blood that is further from the center of the scanner, because the effectiveness of the coil that generates the radiofrequency pulse gets lower the further away you go. In practice, label durations beyond 1 s are hard to achieve. To aid perfusion quantification, methods such as QUIPSS II and Q2TIPS have been developed that saturate, or cut off, the tail end of the bolus at a specified time, thereby defining the label duration (see Box 2.1).

Advantages of pASL:

■ Can be used on clinical scanners without specialist hardware.

■ Relatively robust to magnetic field homogeneity.

■ Labeling efficiency does not depend on blood flow velocity.

■ Relatively low power deposition.

■ Minimal sensitivity to magnetization transfer effects in most recent implementations.

Disadvantages of pASL:

■ Label duration is ill defined unless QUIPSS II or Q2TIPS is used.

■ Label duration is often short compared with cASL (0.6–0.8 s is commonly used), limiting the signal-to-noise ratio (SNR).

■ Greater T_1 decay of the signal compared with cASL since some blood is labeled further from the imaging region and thus takes longer to reach the tissue.

> ### Box 2.1: Restricting label duration in pASL: QUIPSS II and Q2TIPS
>
> One of the potential issues with pASL is an ill-defined label duration. To understand why this is the case, you can imagine a simple scenario in which the labeling region contains arteries that run in straight lines directly upward, toward the brain. In this case, if the thickness of the labeling region is Δz, then, assuming the blood velocity v is constant within the artery, the duration of the resulting bolus of labeled-blood water that is delivered to the brain will be given by $\Delta z / v$. Therefore, the label duration depends on the blood velocity, which is generally unknown and likely to be different in different individuals and even in different arteries in the same individual.
>
> To solve this problem, methods such as QUIPSS II and Q2TIPS were developed that saturate, or cut off, the bolus at a specified time after labeling (TI_1). These techniques remove all magnetization within the labeling region, and therefore all blood flowing into the imaging region after this time does not contribute to the ASL difference signal. Thus, the label duration becomes well defined and equal to TI_1.
>
> It is worth noting that if the time TI_1 is chosen to be too long, then the tail edge of the labeled bolus may have already passed beyond the labeling region when the saturation begins. The true label duration will therefore be shorter than TI_1 and thus unknown. In practice, the combination of typical coil dimensions and arterial flow speeds mean that label durations much beyond 1 s are not achievable with pASL, and thus TI_1 is often set to shorter than this.

2.1.4 Pseudo-continuous ASL (pcASL)

Pseudo-continuous ASL, also known as pulsed-continuous ASL, has much in common with cASL and can be understood in a similar way, as in Figure 2.1. Blood is inverted as it flows through a defined labeling plane, creating a well-defined bolus of labeled blood that can have a long label duration. However, in this case, the long cASL radiofrequency pulse and gradient are broken up into a series of repeating short radiofrequency pulses and associated gradients, which means they can be implemented on standard clinical scanners. In addition, the control condition can be achieved with an almost identical set of radiofrequency pulses and gradients, giving a very well-balanced control.

Advantages of pcASL:

- Can be used on clinical scanners without specialist hardware.
- Well-defined label duration, simplifying perfusion quantification.
- Relatively high labeling efficiency.
- Long label durations are achievable, maximizing SNR.
- Very well-matched control condition
- Suitable for vessel-selective applications (see Box 2.2).

Disadvantages of pcASL:

- Some sensitivity to magnetic field inhomogeneity and blood flow velocity.
- Relatively high power deposition.
- Acoustic noise during the scan can be significant (see Box 2.3).

Box 2.2: Vessel-selective ASL

Rather than labeling all the blood flowing into the brain, it is also possible to use ASL to specifically target individual feeding arteries, allowing visualization of the different vascular territories—the regions of the brain fed by a specific artery. This can be useful for observing phenomena such as compensatory (collateral) blood flow in diseases, when the normal feeding artery is narrowed or blocked, or arterial supply to various lesions. pcASL is well suited to this application, and can be modified either to label individual arteries or to "encode" different combinations of arteries across multiple images, such that the signal arising from each feeding artery can be calculated in post-processing in an SNR-efficient way.

The details of the analysis of the "vessel-encoded" ASL approach are beyond this primer. However, after separation of the signals arising from each artery, the resulting perfusion signals can be processed in an identical manner to conventional ASL data. An example of absolute perfusion and arterial transit time maps resulting from a multi-PLD vessel-encoded pcASL approach are shown in Figure 2.2. The color in the CBF map indicates the arterial origin of the blood signal in each voxel, as shown in the legend.

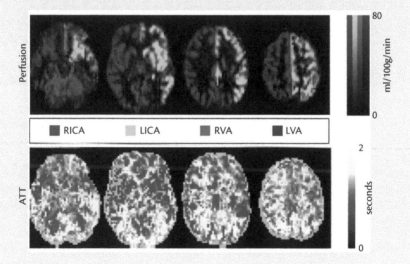

Figure 2.2: Perfusion and ATT images from a vessel-encoded pcASL scan. The perfusion image is color-coded to show the contributions from different arteries feeding the brain. The flow territories can be seen in this image—specific areas of the brain receive blood from specific arteries (of which there are four that supply the majority of brain tissue). Note that the posterior territory is a mixed supply for the two vertebral arteries. (R/LICA: right/left internal carotid artery; R/LVA: right/left vertebral artery).

Box 2.3: **Acoustic noise**

If you have ever been in, or near, an MRI scanner, you will know that they produce a lot of acoustic noise when they are running. However, since pcASL relies on a rapidly repeating series of radiofrequency pulses and gradients, it results in an often loud and high-pitched noise during the labeling period. This is not the case for cASL or pASL. While participants should be wearing effective hearing protection and most are not alarmed by the noise, it is worth bearing in mind that nervous subjects may not be very comfortable with this, particularly if they are not warned about it beforehand!

2.1.5 Labeling summary

Owing to its high SNR efficiency, ability to be run on clinical MRI scanners, well-defined label duration, and well-balanced control condition, pcASL is the recommended labeling scheme for most situations. However, researchers should be aware that the labeling efficiency has some sensitivity to blood flow velocity at the labeling plane, so care should be taken in patient groups with unusually high or low blood velocities or in studies where blood flow velocity may be altered between two conditions (e.g., through administration of a drug).

2.2 Waiting

After the arterial blood has been labeled, we need to wait for that labeled blood to arrive at the tissue before we attempt to measure the perfusion signal. The definition of this waiting period is slightly different between different ASL methods, as shown schematically in Figure 2.3. For cASL or pcASL, labeling is performed for a fixed amount of time (the labeling duration). During this period, blood that has already been labeled starts to flow toward the tissue. At the end of the labeling period, there is a post-labeling delay (PLD) to allow the tail end of the bolus of labeled blood to reach the tissue before an image is acquired.

In pASL, the labeling is nearly instantaneous, and the period of time allowed for this labeled blood to reach the tissue is known as the inversion time (TI, or sometimes TI_2). If a method such as QUIPSS II is used to try to achieve a well-defined label duration, then the time at which it is applied is referred to as TI_1 (see Box 2.1). Since this defines the duration of the bolus of labeled blood, TI_1 is equivalent to the cASL/pcASL labeling duration. The time then available for the tail end of the bolus to reach the tissue before imaging, $TI - TI_1$, is analogous to the cASL/pcASL post-labeling delay.

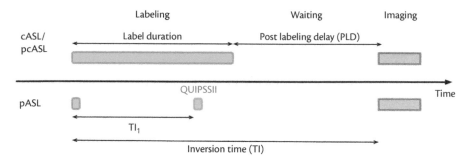

Figure 2.3: Schematic of the ASL pulse sequence timing parameters. The timing and approximate duration of the applications of different radiofrequency fields are shown, including those relating to labeling (blue), imaging (orange), and, for pASL, the QUIPSS II (or Q2TIPS) pulse (green).

2.2.1 How long should we wait?

There are two main factors that determine how long we should wait for labeled blood-water to arrive at the tissue. On the one hand, we want to wait long enough for all of the labeled blood to have had time to traverse the arterial tree and reach the tissue of interest. This not only maximizes the amount of labeled blood that contributes to the ASL signal, but also ensures that the signal we measure is approximately proportional to tissue perfusion (this is discussed in more detail in Chapter 4). On the other hand, the signal difference between labeled and unlabeled blood decays exponentially with characteristic time T_1. Therefore if we wait too long, the ASL signal will be extremely small and difficult to distinguish from any sources of noise in the images.

Based on these two competing factors, the optimum post-labeling delay (PLD, or $TI - TI_1$ for pASL) should be set equal to the longest time expected for the blood to travel from the point of labeling to the tissue, i.e., the longest expected arterial transit time (ATT). This poses a problem though: How do we know beforehand how long the blood will take to arrive at the tissue in any given subject? For healthy volunteers within a particular age range, some experiments can be performed to try to measure this for a particular ASL labeling location. However, in subjects with different ages or with diseases that affect the vasculature, the blood can often be significantly delayed. Some guidance on suitable PLDs for different subjects is given in the ASL consensus paper, see Section 2.8.

2.2.2 Single- versus multi-PLD ASL

A single-delay ASL protocol in which a single PLD or TI is used is simple, easy to implement, and, within a given scan time, allows many averages of each label and control image to be acquired in order to boost the SNR. However, to fulfill the requirement that the PLD is longer than the longest ATT expected in a given group of subjects, a very long PLD must be chosen, which reduces the strength of the ASL signal. In addition, it is difficult to know, even retrospectively, whether the PLD chosen was sufficient to allow the complete arrival of blood to the tissue.

An alternative is to acquire ASL data at multiple delay times, often referred to as multi-PLD or multi-TI data. Once acquired, a kinetic model can be fit to the data (see Chapter 4) to allow the simultaneous estimation of perfusion and ATT. A multi-PLD protocol is therefore less sensitive to differences in ATT across the tissue and across subjects than a single-PLD protocol. An additional benefit is that the restriction on using a long PLD is lifted, so the ASL signal can be sampled earlier when it is stronger, boosting the average signal strength. If some longer PLDs are also included in the protocol, then some sensitivity to delayed blood arrival is still maintained. Finally, ATT may be an interesting physiological parameter in its own right, so a richer set of information can be derived from a multi-delay protocol.

One consideration for the multi-delay approach is that within a given scan time, the number of averages achievable at each PLD reduces in proportion to the number of PLDs to be sampled. Thus, the images formed at each PLD will appear noisier. However, it must be remembered that all of the information, across all the PLDs, is combined during kinetic model fitting, which is akin to collecting more averages at a single PLD, resulting in more robust estimates of perfusion. Another potential disadvantage of multi-PLD protocols is that sampling at earlier time points increases sensitivity to blood signal that still resides within large arterial structures before it has had time to reach the tissue. This can be addressed by trying to remove this signal at the point of acquisition (see Section 2.7) or by including such macrovascular signal within the kinetic model during the fitting process (see Section 4.3).

Further discussion and examples of estimating perfusion using single- and multi-PLD data are given in chapter 4. Some more advanced multi-delay methods are also discussed in Box 2.4.

Box 2.4: Advanced multi-delay ASL methods

Rather than sequentially acquiring ASL data using different PLDs or TIs for different measurements, some alternative strategies have been proposed, shown schematically in Figure 2.4. In "Look-Locker" style acquisitions, which include the QUASAR (quantitative STAR labeling of arterial regions) technique, rather than just acquiring a single image after each ASL labeling or control period, a series of images is obtained for each labeled bolus created. In this manner, the full kinetic curve can be sampled after each ASL preparation, saving a considerable amount of time compared with cycling through the various PLDs on different measurements. However, this must be done cautiously, since the acquisition of the earlier images can significantly reduce the ASL signal remaining in the later images. In addition, the number of slices that can be acquired is determined by the desired temporal resolution (i.e., the spacing of the acquired PLDs), which may limit spatial coverage.

A more recently proposed alternative is time-encoded (also known as Hadamard-encoded) ASL. In this cASL/pcASL technique, the time period prior to image acquisition is broken up into a number of sub-periods or "blocks." Each block can be independently assigned as either "label" or "control," indicating whether the radiofrequency field that induces inversion of blood-water flowing through the labeling plane is on or off. After this preparation period, a single image is acquired. This process is repeated with the blocks set into different combinations of "label" and "control" prior to the acquisition of each image. In this manner, the final ASL signal over a number of separate images contains an encoded pattern as set by the different combinations of blocks in the preparation. This encoding can be decoded in analysis to generate a series of images with different effective PLDs. The main advantage of this approach is that the combination of many images to produce each output image leads to greater averaging of the noise, improving the SNR. However, using a larger number of blocks to improve the temporal resolution also reduces the effective labeling duration of each block, which then reduces the SNR.

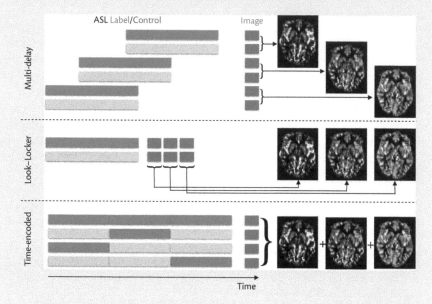

Figure 2.4: Schematic of three different methods for obtaining multi-PLD ASL data. In the conventional multi-delay approach, both label (orange) and control (gray) images are acquired with one PLD before moving on to the next PLD. In the "Look-Locker" approach, multiple images are acquired at different times after a single ASL preparation, each with a different effective PLD. In the time-encoded approach, only a single image is acquired after each ASL preparation period. However, the preparation period is broken up into a series of "blocks," which are set to be either labeling or control, in different combinations across a number of acquisitions. In this example, the preparation period is split into three blocks of equal length. The first image is acquired where blood is labeled during all three blocks. The second image is acquired when a control is applied during the first and third blocks, while labeling occurs during the second block. Combining images with different labeling and control combinations during these blocks in post-processing allows the calculation of how much labeled blood signal arises from blood labeled during each block. Since each block occurs at a different delay prior to imaging, perfusion images at different effective PLDs are generated.

2.3 Readout

After we have labeled the incoming blood and waited for it to arrive at the tissue, we need to acquire an image of the brain. There are a wide variety of options for image acquisition, or *readout*. Here we will briefly cover some of the more popular methods and some of their advantages and disadvantages.

2.3.1 2D multi-slice versus 3D readouts

A schematic showing the difference between 2D multi-slice and 3D readout methods is shown in Figure 2.5. In 2D multi-slice methods, all imaging data from a single slice is acquired before moving on to the next slice. In this example, the lowest (most inferior) slice is acquired first before sequentially acquiring higher (more superior) slices. In contrast, for 3D readouts, the signal from the entire brain is acquired simultaneously. Note that the 3D readouts used in ASL are often very different from those used in other applications, such as structural imaging. For those more familiar with MRI methods, some discussion of the differences is given in Box 2.5.

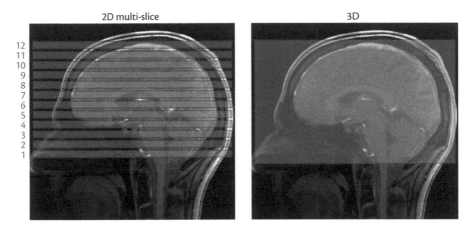

Figure 2.5: 2D multi-slice versus 3D readout schemes. In a 2D approach the slices are acquired sequentially, often for ASL in ascending order, whereas for 3D the full 3D volume is acquired simultaneously.

Box 2.5: **3D readouts for ASL**

3D readouts are often used in structural imaging because of their high SNR, minimal distortions, and ability to produce high-resolution images with isotropic resolution. However, the 3D readouts used for ASL are often very different from those used in structural imaging. Since labeling the blood and waiting for it to arrive in the brain takes up a considerable amount of time, it is important that as much imaging data is acquired after each ASL preparation as possible to avoid having to repeat the process many times for each image being reconstructed. In addition, every time the magnetization is excited to allow an image to be generated, the ASL signal is reduced. For this reason, 3D readouts for ASL typically rely on using a single excitation pulse after each ASL preparation, rather than the thousands of excitation pulses often used in structural imaging. This excitation pulse is followed by the rapid acquisition of as much imaging data as possible. It is possible to acquire enough data for a full 3D volume after a single excitation pulse, although, as discussed in the text, this takes some time during which the signal is decaying exponentially (according to the T_2 of the tissue), which can lead to blurring artifacts.

There are a number of implications from the choice of 2D versus 3D readouts:

- **Slice timing**: For 2D multi-slice readouts, each slice is acquired at a different time after the ASL preparation. This means that the effective PLD of each slice is different and must be accounted for in the analysis. In addition, it is more difficult to achieve effective background suppression (discussed in Section 2.4) across all the slices. For 3D readouts, the image contrast is effectively fixed at one point in time, giving a consistent PLD and background suppression across the brain.

- **SNR**: 3D readouts generally have higher SNR than 2D readouts.

- **Blurring**: Once the signal has been produced, it begins to decay. In 2D readouts, the signal from each slice is acquired separately, so signal decay during the acquisition of a single slice has little impact. However, it takes much longer to acquire all the data necessary to reconstruct a full 3D image, so signal decay during this time can become significant. For most 3D imaging methods used with ASL, this manifests as a blurring of signals across the different slices, effectively reducing the spatial resolution in the slice direction.

- **Segmentation**: To avoid significant blurring problems, one option is to "segment" the 3D readout (also referred to as "multi-shot" readouts). This means that only some fraction of the information required to reconstruct the whole brain is acquired after each ASL preparation. This reduces the readout time and therefore the blurring artifact. However, it also means that data acquired over multiple ASL preparations must be combined before an image can be reconstructed, considerably increasing the scan time required to produce a given number of images.

- **Motion sensitivity**: ASL relies on the subtraction of label and control images, and is therefore very sensitive to motion. Post-processing can be used to align images after the acquisition to correct for gross subject motion (see Section 3.1). However, this approach fails for motion that happens *during* the acquisition of information for a single volume. This problem is exacerbated for segmented (multi-shot) 3D readouts, where information about a single volume is acquired over multiple ASL preparations. Significant motion during a 2D multi-slice readout can lead to distortion of the shape of the brain and also "spin-history" effects, which can cause a loss of signal if part of the brain that was imaged in a previous slice moves to a location within a subsequently acquired slice (i.e., the same brain region is unintentionally imaged multiple times within the same volume). Such effects are extremely difficult to remove in post-processing. Single-shot 3D imaging methods are perhaps the least sensitive to these effects.

2.3.2 Commonly used readout schemes

A wide variety of readout approaches have been combined with ASL, all with their advantages and disadvantages. Some commonly used 2D multi-slice readouts include the following:

- **Echo-planar imaging (EPI)**: Also widely used in other applications, such as fMRI and diffusion imaging, EPI is a very efficient 2D multi-slice method in which a single slice can be acquired very rapidly (typically within ~50 ms). While very efficient, it does suffer from signal dropout and distortion artifacts in regions with poor magnetic field homogeneity (e.g., around the sinuses and ear canals). Spin-echo EPI is a variant that helps to reduce signal dropout artifacts, but adds to the acquisition time, so is less frequently used for ASL. A more advanced version of EPI, multi-band EPI, is discussed in Box 2.6.

■ **Spiral**: This method is similar to EPI, but the data is acquired in a slightly different way. Advantages over EPI include the ability to achieve a very short echo time (TE), which helps to reduce signal dropout artifacts, and the more rapid acquisition of each slice for similar imaging parameters. However, image reconstruction is more complex and, rather than the image distortions seen with EPI in regions of poor magnetic field homogeneity, spiral readouts lead to image blurring, which is difficult to correct in post-processing (see Section 3.2).

Both EPI and spiral readouts have related 3D readouts that are also commonly used, both having the benefits and drawbacks of 3D methods mentioned in Section 2.3.1:

■ **3D-gradient and spin echo (3D-GRASE)**: This method has much in common with spin-echo EPI: signal dropout artifacts are minimal, but EPI-like distortions are still present.

■ **3D rapid acquisition with relaxation enhancement (RARE) stack-of-spirals**: This is a 3D extension of the spiral method, in much the same way as 3D-GRASE is a 3D extension of EPI. It has minimal signal dropout, but suffers from in-plane blurring in regions of magnetic field inhomogeneity, in the same way as spiral imaging, which is difficult to correct in post-processing. However, one potential advantage over 3D-GRASE is that the readout is more rapid, which reduces the total readout duration and therefore the through-slice blurring.

Box 2.6: **Multi-band EPI**

Another readout scheme that is rapidly gaining in popularity for fMRI and diffusion imaging is multi-band (MB) EPI. Some recent ASL implementations are also using this technique. In essence, it is very similar to standard EPI imaging, but rather than imaging only a single 2D slice at a time, multiple 2D slices are imaged simultaneously and then separated out in image reconstruction by leveraging the additional spatial information provided by using a multi-channel head coil array. An important implication for an ASL dataset acquired using multi-band EPI is that the PLD and background suppression variation with slice number will now follow a more complicated pattern (neither sequential nor interleaved) determined by how many and which slices were acquired simultaneously (e.g., slices 1, 5, 9, etc. could be acquired at the same time, with slices 2, 6, 10, etc. at another time, and so on).

2.3.3 Readout parameter considerations

ASL is intrinsically a low-SNR technique. It is important to be aware of this when choosing your imaging parameters, since these have a significant impact on the SNR of the resulting images. The optimal parameter choices will depend on the readout scheme being used, the imaging time available, the field strength of the scanner, the size of the perfusion differences that are of interest for your study, and many other factors. Some broad considerations on readout parameter choices include the following:

- **Spatial resolution**: SNR scales with voxel volume, so a seemingly small change in the voxel volume, for example, 4 mm × 4 mm × 4 mm to 3 mm × 3 mm × 3 mm, will lead to the SNR being reduced by a large factor (2.4 times in this case). This has a big impact on a low-SNR technique like ASL. SNR can be regained by increasing the number of repeated measurements (averages) acquired, but the SNR only scales with the square root of the number of averages. In this example, the scan time would have to be increased by a factor of $2.4^2 = 5.6$ to maintain the SNR at the same level (e.g., a 5-minute scan would become a 28-minute scan!). Using a lower spatial resolution (larger voxels) also decreases the time required for the readout period. However, be aware that using very low spatial resolution will clearly impair the ability to localize the perfusion signal to precise brain regions, as well as exacerbating partial volume effects (see Chapter 6), and can also increase signal dropout artifacts that occur in regions with poor magnetic field homogeneity (e.g., near the sinuses or ear canals). Typically, higher spatial resolution can be achieved at higher field strengths, but at 3 T, voxel sizes of 4 mm × 4 mm × 4 mm or 3.5 mm × 3.5 mm × 5 mm are reasonable.

- **Echo time (TE)**: The echo time determines how much signal decay occurs before the image is acquired. Unlike BOLD fMRI, there is no need to use a long TE in ASL, so minimizing the echo time will help improve SNR and minimize signal dropout artifacts for non-spin-echo techniques. Spiral-based readouts intrinsically have low echo times. For EPI-based methods, keeping the spatial resolution low will help keep the TE low, but a technique known as "partial Fourier" or "half-scan" can also be used. With this method, the TE can be reduced, improving the SNR, although this is often accompanied by a small amount of image blurring.

- **Parallel imaging**: This technique reduces the time required for the readout by using the spatial information from multiple coils (also used in multi-band EPI, but in a different way) to reduce the number of samples of the MRI signal that need to be acquired. This can help to minimize TE and reduce the total readout duration, which also reduces through-slice blurring in 3D methods. However, this comes at the cost of SNR, and some additional scan time is required for the parallel imaging to be calibrated, which may often outweigh the potential benefits.

- **Artifacts**: As mentioned already, various readout parameters will impact on the potential for image artifacts. For example, large voxels (or thick slices) and long echo times will exacerbate signal dropout, longer readout durations will result in more severe image distortions (for EPI-based methods) or blurring artifacts (for spiral-based methods) as well as through-slice blurring (for 3D methods), and motion artifacts will be more problematic for segmented 3D readouts.

2.3.4 Readout summary

There are a variety of different readout methods, each with their own advantages and disadvantages. The optimal choice is likely to depend on the imaging time available, the cohort of subjects (e.g. are they likely to move during the scan?) and the expected perfusion signal differences of interest, along with the local availability of different sequences. In practice, what you have available to you will be determined by whoever is providing your MRI sequences: you can often get a clue to what version of ASL you have as explained in Box 2.7. Irrespective of what ASL variant you have or choose, piloting a given protocol is key to ensuring that sufficient image quality is obtained under the restrictions for a given study.

Box 2.7: Which version of ASL do I have?

On your scanner, the ASL pulse sequence you are using may have a rather opaque name, like "ep2d_picore." Looking through the various options within the protocol might help to clarify which version of ASL is being run. If there is any doubt, we thoroughly recommend clarifying with your scanner vendor representative, or whoever provided the pulse sequence, exactly which flavor of ASL you have and the readout scheme being used. However, as a rough guide, cASL or pcASL sequences will often have "CASL" or "PCASL" in the name. On the other hand, there are many different versions of PASL. Some of the most common are EPISTAR, PICORE, and FAIR. The other parts of the sequence name often refer to the readout scheme being used. For example, "ep2d" refers to 2D multi-slice EPI, one of the many readout options possible. From an analysis perspective, it is important to understand which type of ASL is being used, the labeling parameters (such as the labeling duration and post-labeling delay), and the type of readout, since these all have implications for the analysis methods used to quantify perfusion.

2.4 Background suppression

In many MRI-based techniques, it is often desirable to maximize the tissue signal that is measured in order to be able to visualize it more clearly above the ever-present noise. ASL is a rather unusual case in this regard, since signal arising from the brain tissue itself is not of interest. In fact, we aim to completely remove any contributions it makes using label–control subtraction. Any changes in the tissue signal between the label and control conditions will be interpreted as "perfusion" signal, biasing our measurements. We therefore aim to ensure that the tissue signal is as similar as possible between label and control conditions, for example by ensuring that magnetization transfer effects are the same in both cases (see Section 2.1).

Since the tissue signal should remain unchanged between label and control, it is often called the *static tissue*, to distinguish it from signal arising from labeled blood-water that has been delivered to the voxel. However, the tissue signal may also fluctuate owing to physiological processes (e.g., with the cardiac or respiratory cycles) and to gross subject motion, which can never be perfectly corrected for in post-processing. Such fluctuations can be significant compared with the small perfusion signal that we are attempting to measure. ASL image quality can therefore be significantly improved by the application of background suppression: that is, we aim to reduce the signal arising from the brain tissue without adversely affecting the perfusion signal. As long as the background suppression is consistent between label and control conditions, the average tissue will still be removed by the subtraction process, but fluctuations in the tissue signal will be considerably reduced. Implementation of background suppression is discussed in more detail in Box 2.8.

Box 2.8: Implementation of background suppression

One simple method to reduce the static tissue signal is to use a "saturation" pulse. This removes any signal present within the imaging region at the time the pulse is applied. If this pulse is applied after labeled blood has begun to accumulate in the brain, then this signal will also be destroyed. Therefore, "pre-saturation" is often applied to remove the static tissue signal before labeling commences. "Post-saturation" is also possible in pASL, since, just after the short labeling pulse, the blood has not yet had time to flow into the imaging region. This not the case with cASL/pcASL, where labeled blood flows into the imaging region during the labeling period.

However, pre- or post-saturation alone typically does not result in effective background suppression, since, as soon as the saturation has been performed, the tissue will begin to recover back toward equilibrium according to its longitudinal relaxation time constant, T_1. Since the labeling period and post-labeling delay are often quite long compared with typical T_1 values found in the brain, this still leaves significant tissue signal present at the time of imaging. Background suppression can be considerably improved through the introduction of additional inversion pulses, often combined with pre- or post-saturation. These are similar to the inversion pulses used to label the blood in pASL techniques, but for background suppression they are applied to the imaging region and can be timed in such a way as to leave very little static tissue signal when imaging commences.

But what effect does this have on the blood-water signal? Blood-water that will contribute to the ASL signal starts in the neck and therefore does not experience the pre- or post-saturation, since this is only applied to the imaging region. It therefore only experiences the inversion pulses. Although the blood-water signal is affected by these pulses, it turns out that the difference in the signal between label and control conditions does not change, and thus the ASL contrast is maintained.

2.4.1 Implications for analysis

Effective background suppression undoubtedly greatly increases the image quality in ASL data. It is particularly important for segmented 3D readout schemes, where small differences in the static tissue signal between "shots" can lead to significant artifacts. However, it does have a number of implications for post-processing of the data:

- **Slice variation**: For 3D readouts, the image contrast is effectively fixed at one point in time, meaning that background suppression can be timed to give effective suppression at this moment. However, for 2D multi-slice readouts, each slice is acquired at a different point in time. The static tissue will continue recovering during this time, meaning that slices acquired later will have less effective background suppression. An example of this effect is shown in Figure 2.6. This can potentially cause problems with registration and motion correction (see Chapter 3), since the tissue signal varies over space. This may be particularly problematic for multi-band readout schemes, where several slices are acquired simultaneously.

- **Motion correction**: In theory, background suppression could be so effective as to remove the static tissue signal altogether. This would appear to be excellent from the perspective

Poor tissue suppression

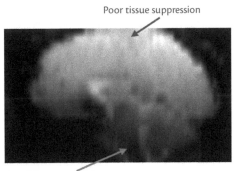

Good tissue suppression

Figure 2.6: Variation in background suppression with slice using a 2D multi-slice readout. A sagittal view of this data set is shown, where the bottom-most (inferior) slices (horizontal cross-sections in this view, as the slice plane was axial) were acquired first and the topmost (superior) slices were acquired last. The background suppression is therefore most effective inferiorly and gets poorer in more superior slices.

of reducing subtraction artifacts due to motion. However, head motion will also affect the perfusion signal, and we wish to be able to correct for this in preprocessing: a process that relies upon aligning the images (see Section 3.1). If the background signal of the brain has been removed too effectively, this correction becomes difficult and may be so inaccurate that it starts introducing artifacts into the label–control subtracted images. This, as well as the danger of inversion of the static tissue signal itself (see Box 2.9), are good reasons for not being too aggressive with the specification of background suppression.

■ **Inversion efficiency**: If inversion pulses are utilized for background suppression, then for ideal pulses the perfusion signal is unaffected. In reality, the pulses are imperfect and lead to a small loss of perfusion signal. Ideally, the efficiency of the pulses should be measured and used to correct the inversion efficiency that is applied in CBF estimation. For example, if two global inversion pulses were used and each had a 95% efficiency, then the inversion efficiency used for quantification should be multiplied by $0.95^2 = 0.9025$.

Box 2.9: **Inverted static tissue**

Most MR images show the "magnitude" (strength) of the signal at each point in space. They are therefore not sensitive to whether the signal is inverted or not. If aggressive background suppression is used, it is possible that the static tissue signal may be inverted at the image acquisition time. This would be problematic for processing ASL magnitude images, since we generally assume that inflowing labeled (inverted) blood reduces the total signal, and therefore subtracting a label image from a control image gives positive perfusion signal. However, if the tissue signal is already inverted, then inverted blood will *add to, not subtract from*, the magnitude of the signal. The control minus label subtraction will then result in negative perfusion signal. It is therefore advisable to ensure that the static tissue signal is uninverted at the imaging time if conventional magnitude image processing is to be performed.

2.5 Calibration scans

The subtraction of control and label ASL scans yields a perfusion-weighted image, but the scaling of such images is somewhat arbitrary. The numbers produced in each voxel will depend on the type of scanner being used, the readout technique employed, the radiofrequency coil used to receive the signal, how the subject is positioned within the coil, and a whole range of other factors. In order to express the perfusion signal in meaningful units, we need some sort of calibration that tells us how to scale the signal appropriately. As we discussed in Chapter 1, this is done by acquiring a separate calibration image in which all ASL labeling and background suppression have been turned off. A long period between image acquisitions (the repetition time, TR, typically 6–10 s) is also used so that the image is dominated by the amount of water in the tissue and not other properties: a proton-density-weighted image. In some acquisition schemes, the calibration image may be acquired as part of the same ASL scan, or it may be a separate image that you need to ask for. Knowing which scan in a series is the calibration image is very important and is not consistent between sequences. The possibilities of how the different images may be ordered in the acquisition (known as "sequence looping") are discussed further in Box 2.10.

Box 2.10: Sequence looping

When it comes to analyzing your ASL data, it is of course important to know which volume of your data corresponds to which ASL preparation. There are many different ASL implementations that may loop through the various combinations of label and control conditions and different PLDs for multi-PLD experiments. In some sequences, different PLDs may be acquired as separate scans, whereas in others they may be interleaved across the acquired volumes. Label conditions may be acquired before control conditions, or vice versa. In addition, a calibration scan may be acquired as the first (or last) volume of the scan, and there may be a single volume or multiple volumes used for the calibration.

It is therefore important to understand how the implementation you are using loops through all these various options to avoid errors in the data analysis. It is also wise to look at your acquired raw data, not only to assess the image quality and degree of motion, but also to make sure that the sequence is looping in the way you expect. If background suppression is being used, then typically images acquired at different PLDs will have slightly different background suppression, and therefore you will be able to see a visual difference in the tissue signal (and perhaps contrast) between different PLDs. Calibration images should appear much more intense, since the tissue signal is not being suppressed (unless a different "gain" factor has been applied: see Box 5.4), and often the contrast between tissue types is more evident. It should also be apparent whether an in-built correction for receive coil sensitivity has been applied. If it has, then the signal strength from a given tissue type across the image should have roughly the same intensity. If the signal close to the receive coil is more intense, then a correction has not been applied, and this must be accounted for the in the analysis.

2.6 Receive-coil sensitivity correction

One other factor that needs to be accounted for is the variable sensitivity of the radiofrequency receive coil being used. Most modern scanners use multi-channel receive (head) coil arrays that are more sensitive to signals near the edges of the brain and less so in the center. If not properly accounted for, the perfusion signal could appear to be artificially larger around the edges of the brain. This is inherently accounted for if voxelwise calibration is used (see Chapter 5), but for other calibration methods it must be corrected for in other ways.

Some scanners allow receive coil sensitivity variations (also known as "bias fields") to be estimated and corrected as part of the acquisition, so that the resulting images are not affected by these variations (see Figure 2.7). If all the ASL and calibration images are acquired with this correction turned on, then no additional post-processing is necessary. If not, then it is possible to estimate the receive-coil sensitivity pattern by acquiring calibration images with and without the correction and dividing one by the other. If no such correction is available on the scanner, an alternative is to acquire one calibration image with the head receive coil as usual and another using the body coil, which is built into most clinical scanners. The body coil is not typically used as a receive coil since the resulting SNR is low, but it does have the advantage of having very little variation in its sensitivity across the brain. Therefore, dividing the image acquired with the head coil by the image acquired with the body coil also produces an estimate of the receive coil sensitivity. Once such an estimate has been obtained, it can be applied to the other ASL data to remove this source of bias.

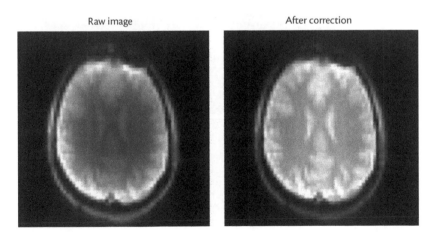

Figure 2.7: Receive-coil sensitivity: examples of images acquired using a multi-channel receive coil without (left) and with (right) coil sensitivity correction applied at the point of acquisition. Note the significant impact of the coil sensitivity, and the much more uniform appearance of the image after correction.

2.7 Arterial artifacts

In much of the discussion of ASL, it is assumed that the blood signal we measure arrives at the voxel and then perfuses the tissue in that voxel. In reality, of course, there are arterial vessels that carry the labeled blood throughout the brain, and using ASL we can observe the labeled blood-water while it is still in the arteries. In fact, ASL has been used to generate angiographic images of the arteries themselves and thereby to measure blood flow rates. However, for perfusion imaging, these arteries will result in ASL signal in voxels where the labeled blood-water is actually destined for elsewhere in the brain and thus should not be contributing to our measure of perfusion, as we discussed in Chapter 1. This is particularly apparent if a short PLD or TI is used, so imaging occurs before the labeled blood has had time to reach the tissue, as shown in Figure 2.8.

There are three main possibilities for dealing with this issue: the first is to use a single-delay approach with a long PLD in the hope that all of the labeled blood has had time to reach the tissue. However, as mentioned previously, this leads to a low SNR efficiency and no information about the arterial transit time, and does not guarantee that no arterial signal will be present if there is delayed blood arrival. This could be particularly problematic in more elderly subjects or in individuals with specific vascular pathologies, such as stenosis. In these cases, an even longer PLD might be required, resulting in an even lower SNR. It is certainly always a good idea to inspect single PLD ASL perfusion images for signs of arterial blood signal, such as those seen in Figure 2.8.

The second approach to correcting for arterial blood signal contributions is to accept that there will be a contribution to the signal in the images and try to model it in analysis so that it does not confound the estimation of tissue perfusion; this is discussed in more detail in Section 4.3. The third option is to try to remove the arterial signal at the point of acquisition, a process known as "flow suppression" or "flow crushing," see Box 2.11. A variant of ASL that you might meet that makes particular use of flow suppression, QUASAR, is described in more detail in Box 2.12.

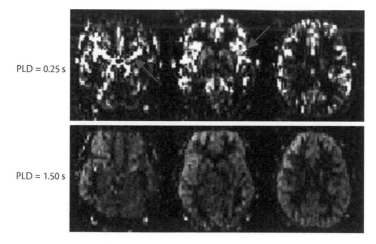

PLD = 0.25 s

PLD = 1.50 s

Figure 2.8: Example pcASL data acquired with a short PLD (0.25 s, top) and a long PLD (1.50 s, bottom). Three example slices are shown, with the leftmost image being the most inferior and the rightmost image being the most superior. Note the large signal contributions from labeled blood within arteries at the shorter PLD (red arrows). At a PLD of 1.50 s, these arterial features have gone, since all the labeled blood-water has had time to reach the tissue.

Box 2.11: **Flow suppression**

Suppression of ASL signal arising from arteries can be achieved by inserting an additional pair of gradient pulses during the image acquisition process. These are identical in principle to the gradient pulses used to generate contrast in diffusion-weighted imaging: if a voxel contains water that is moving at a range of velocities (as is the case in arterial structures), then the gradient pulses cause these signals to cancel each other out, greatly reducing the arterial signal. For diffusion imaging, very large gradients are required to make the acquisition sensitive to motion on the microscopic scale. For flow suppression, blood is typically moving at speeds of the order of centimeters per second, so much smaller gradients can be used.

The advantage of this approach is that, in theory, very little arterial signal is present in the resulting images, so only the tissue signal needs to be considered in the subsequent analysis. However, the additional gradient pulses required take some time to play out, meaning that the echo time (TE) has to be extended. As mentioned in Section 2.3, in general we want to minimize TE in ASL to maximize the SNR and reduce sensitivity to signal dropout artifacts, so adding flow suppression gradients is detrimental in this way. In addition, the flow-suppressing gradients must be applied in a particular direction. Only blood flowing in this direction will be optimally suppressed, whereas blood flowing orthogonally to this direction will not be affected. Suppression in the inferior–superior direction is often chosen, since blood tends to travel upward, but there are significant arterial segments that run within the axial plane that would not be affected by such gradients. Therefore, it is likely that some arterial signal will still be present in the resulting images (Figure 2.9).

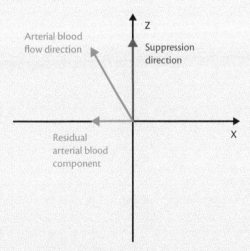

Figure 2.9: Arterial suppression is normally applied in the inferior–superior direction, commonly labeled the *z*-direction. Any arterial blood flow not perfectly aligned in this direction will not be perfectly suppressed, and a component will remain, as illustrated here on the *x*-axis perpendicular to the suppression direction, which will lead to some arterial signal appearing in the ASL data.

> **Box 2.12: QUASAR**
>
> Quantitative STAR labeling of arterial regions (QUASAR), is a Look-Locker pASL method that repeatedly images the brain after a single ASL preparation to generate many images at different TIs. However, QUASAR also involves the acquisition of two ASL data sets: one with flow-crushing gradients applied and one without. Both data sets contain ASL signal within the tissue, but only the non-crushed data set contains arterial signal. Therefore, the subtraction of the two isolates just the arterial signal, which can be used to estimate a local arterial input function (see Chapter 4). This can then be used to quantify perfusion without making assumptions about the shape of the bolus of labeled blood, potentially accounting more accurately for effects such as dispersion. The processing of this kind of data is described in more detail in Box 4.13.

2.8 Consensus paper recommendations

The ISMRM Perfusion Study Group and the European Consortium for ASL in Dementia produced a joint consensus paper in 2015 describing a recommended implementation of ASL for perfusion imaging in clinical applications (see Further reading). In brief, the main recommendations are as follows:

- **Labeling**: pcASL with a label duration of 1800 ms.
- **Waiting**: A single PLD of 1800 ms in healthy subjects under 70 years and 2000 ms in patients or subjects over 70 years (separate recommendations for children are also given).
- **Readout**: A segmented 3D readout (without flow suppression gradients).
- **Background suppression**: Pre-saturation followed by two inversion pulses.
- **Calibration image**: Separately acquired image without background suppression and with a long TR.
- **Perfusion calculation**: Performed using a simplified model, as described in Box 1.3, using voxelwise calibration that corrects for receive-coil sensitivity.

If these recommendations are followed, then good quality ASL data should be obtained. However, it is worth remembering that these guidelines were designed to provide a simple protocol, with straightforward perfusion quantification for a range of clinical settings. Therefore, the optimal protocol for a given research study may well differ from these guidelines. For example, multi-PLD ASL was not recommended as the default protocol, owing to its increased complexity, but its use was encouraged, particularly for those who wish to achieve more precise perfusion quantification and/or for those who are interested in estimating the ATT.

In research studies, where complex analyses are often performed as standard across a range of imaging modalities, the increased complexity of a multi-PLD protocol is unlikely to be a concern. For studies where significant motion is expected, a single-shot 3D or multi-slice 2D readout might produce more reliable data than a segmented 3D readout. Therefore, when designing an ASL protocol, the consensus paper recommendations are a good place to start, but researchers should feel free to explore a range of options, taking all the factors for their particular situation into account and testing their choices in practice with pilot data.

SUMMARY

- There are many different methods for acquiring ASL data, all with their advantages and disadvantages.
- For labeling, pcASL is generally the recommended option owing to its high SNR and the ability to achieve long label durations, but in some cases alternative methods may be more suitable.
- pcASL labeling efficiency has some dependence on blood flow velocity at the labeling plane, so researchers performing studies comparing groups that may have different blood flow velocities, or using drugs that may manipulate blood flow rates, should be aware of this.
- Single-PLD ASL is simple to perform but is sensitive to delays in blood arrival unless a very long PLD is chosen, which reduces SNR.
- Multi-PLD ASL allows the estimation and correction for the ATT, but requires more complex post-processing.
- For the readout, 3D sequences allow more efficient background suppression and yield higher SNR, but can suffer from through-slice blurring, and segmented methods are potentially more sensitive to motion artifacts.
- Effective background suppression is very important for achieving high quality ASL images, but the effects must be considered in subsequent analysis.

- The consensus paper recommendations give a robust and simple protocol, particularly for routine clinical applications, but the optimal protocol for specific research studies may differ from these guidelines.

FURTHER READING

- Alsop, D. C., Detre, J. A., Golay, X., Günther, M., Hendrikse, J., Hernandez-Garcia, L., et al. (2015). Recommended implementation of arterial spin-labeled perfusion MRI for clinical applications: A consensus of the ISMRM Perfusion Study Group and the European Consortium for ASL in Dementia. *Magnetic Resonance in Medicine*, 73(1), 102–116.
    - *This ASL "white paper," or "consensus paper," was recommended reading for the previous chapter, it gives a very good summary of the various ASL methods that are available, and it provides recommendations for a simple ASL protocol for routine clinical applications.*

■ Wong, E. C. (2013). New developments in arterial spin labeling pulse sequences. *NMR in Biomedicine, 26*(8), 887–891.

   ■ *This review article gives a nice brief overview of some more advanced ASL methods that we have not had time to cover here. These include methods that allow blood to be labeled based on its velocity rather than its location, mapping of vascular territories, and methods for estimating the oxygen extraction fraction in the brain.*

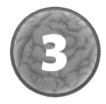

Preprocessing

In this chapter, we consider a number of common analysis steps that are applied to ASL data before quantification of perfusion. These are largely used to remove or reduce artifacts in the data, such as those arising from motion or distortions associated with the readout used. An essential preprocessing step for ASL analysis that we have already met is label–control subtraction, and we will not discuss that further here, except to note that, as we will see, there can be important interactions between subtraction and other preprocessing that you need to be aware of.

3.1 Motion correction

Like all MRI methods, ASL is susceptible to motion, and thus some form of motion correction is often advisable as a preprocessing step, although there are challenges specific to ASL data that can mean it is hard to achieve good correction. The main option for motion correction is the same as that widely used for other functional MRI data: namely to perform registration between the individual volumes using rigid-body (six degrees of freedom) transformations. Common motion correction methods are covered in more detail in the primer in this series "Introduction to Neuroimaging Analysis."

The most noticeable source of error introduced by motion into ASL data arises in the label–control subtraction. Subtle head motion between volumes can give rise to voxel differences that, when two volumes are subtracted from each other, can be as large as, if not larger than, the perfusion signal itself. This is often most visible around the edge of the brain, but is potentially problematic wherever there is significant contrast in the raw data. It is thus important that motion correction be applied before label–control subtraction. The biggest drawback of motion correction is that interpolation is involved in the registration-based correction approach, which itself can lead to subtraction artifacts. It also cannot "undo" the different partial volume effects that will occur when the head moves in relation to the sampling grid of the final images (see Chapter 6).

Subtraction errors arising from motion are also a further motivation for background suppression (see Section 2.4); reducing the static tissue signal and making it more uniform will reduce subtraction artifacts whether they originate from motion or are physiological in origin. While background suppression will reduce motion artifacts, it will, in turn, make motion correction more difficult, since it removes the contrast that the registration process uses to align different volumes accurately. Intuitively, two pictures with faint edges will be harder to align to each other than two with clear, bright edges. Thus, a good background suppression scheme should not be too aggressive and should leave enough static tissue signal for motion correction. Motion correction on multi-PLD data can offer extra challenges because the intensity of the background-suppressed images can vary with the PLD, although common motion correction algorithms should be able to cope with this. Subtle effects have been observed with 2D readouts, where different slices are acquired at different PLDs (see Section 2.3), with later slices typically having poorer background suppression. This can lead to quite a dominant inferior-superior variation in signal intensity, which varies across PLDs: this can interact with the motion correction to cause artificial shifting of the imaging volume in the inferior–superior direction.

Overall, it pays to attempt motion correction of a dataset and then examine the *label–control subtracted images* to look for obvious artifacts, as is done in Example Box 3.1. Often, artifacts are most prominent in only a fraction of volumes, owing to large motion at specific times in the scan. One effective strategy to deal with these artifacts can be to remove this subset of volumes before further processing. This might be particularly relevant where motion has occurred during the readout and thus cannot be corrected for by registration-based motion correction. This can be done manually or automatically, as methods have been developed that judge which volumes to remove. These methods use motion information derived from the registration process and assess whether removal of volumes identified as being at points of large motion improves the overall estimation of the perfusion image, for example, by examining the variance on the estimated perfusion values.

Example Box 3.1: Motion correction of pcASL data

We can revisit the data from the examples in Chapter 1 and see what difference motion correction makes. Note that this data was acquired in a compliant and well-rehearsed volunteer, so we are not expecting the motion to be substantial. Figure 3.1 shows individual difference images from specific volumes before and after motion correction, where some motion corruption is visible before correction, manifesting visually as artifacts around the rim of the brain. Note that the motion correction has reduced the artifacts arising from subtraction, but there is still evidence of an effect even after correction.

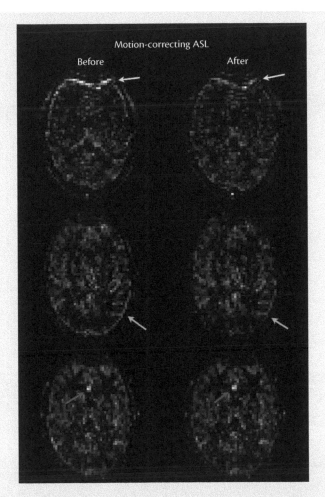

Figure 3.1: Three selected difference images (rows) from the dataset introduced in the examples in Chapter 1, showing images before (left) and after (right) motion correction. The green arrow shows there is less of a rim enhancement after motion correction. Although motion correction does not undo image distortions (yellow arrows) or large-vessel contamination (red arrows), it does help reduce the influence of artifacts arising from them in the subtracted images.

Figure 3.2 shows the mean perfusion-weighted images before and after motion correction. Since the motion in this case was minimal, the visual difference after averaging 30 different pairs is subtle. But this difference largely manifests itself around the edges of the brain, as can be seen by calculating the difference between the two cases as shown in Figure 3.2.

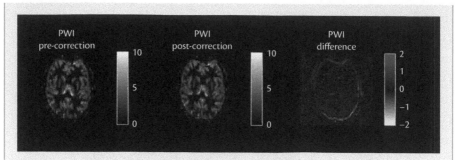

Figure 3.2: Comparison of the perfusion-weighted image before (left) and after (center) motion correction for the dataset introduced in Chapter 1, along with the difference between the two (right).

As we have already noted, motion can be more problematic in data without background suppression. Figure 3.3 shows the perfusion-weighted image produced from a very similar dataset to that in Figure 3.2, only this time no background suppression was applied. The motion errors are more substantial in this case (although direct quantitative comparison with Figure 3.2 is not precise, since the overall scaling in the data is slightly different and the motion will be different in this subject, but still small when examined by eye). Not only is the edge of brain highlighted in the difference between data that has been motion-corrected with that which has not, but also features within the brain including the ventricles and even the cortical folding pattern appear to be contributing.

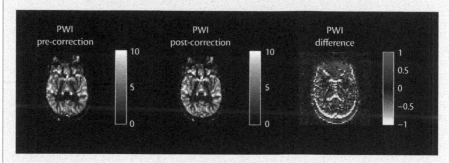

Figure 3.3: Comparison of the perfusion-weighted image before (left) and after (center) motion correction in a dataset without background suppression (but otherwise using parameters similar to the example in Chapter 1), along with the difference between the two (right).

On the primer website, you will find both of the datasets shown here and also instructions on how to perform motion correction and examine the difference it makes on the data and the final computed perfusion image.

3.2 Distortion correction

ASL data acquired using echo planar imaging (EPI), including the 3D-GRASE readout, will also suffer from distortions common to all EPI-based techniques, and methods that are used to correct for these in other MRI applications (e.g., BOLD fMRI) can be applied to ASL. One option is to acquire the calibration image twice with opposite phase-encode directions (e.g., anterior–posterior then posterior–anterior) and use this to correct for distortions in both the calibration image and in the main ASL data series; this is the method used in Example Box 3.2. Alternatively, where a field map has been collected (possibly as part of another acquisition within the same session, such as a diffusion or BOLD fMRI scan) this can be used to correct for the distortions. For more information on distortion correction, see the primer in this series "Introduction to Neuroimaging Analysis." Distortion associated with spiral readouts, however, cannot be corrected for in the same way.

Example Box 3.2: EPI distortion correction

Once again, we can revisit the data from the examples in Chapter 1, but now apply distortion correction. The dataset includes two calibration images: one with phase encoding in the anterior–posterior direction, which matches the main ASL data, and also a separate calibration image with phase encoding posterior–anterior. These two images can be seen in Figure 3.4; notice that the biggest effect is visible at the anterior part of the brain. We have chosen to view a slightly lower slice in this figure, compared with those we looked at in Chapter 1, since the distortion is more obvious where the field inhomogeneity is bigger, nearer to the air-filled sinuses. Using these two images, a field map can be estimated and this then used to combine the two calibration images into one corrected image, on the right of Figure 3.4. We can also apply the same correction to the main ASL data to correct for the (identical) distortion that will be present there too. Note that we have only acquired two versions of the calibration image, we did not have to duplicate the main ASL acquisition and so the extra acquisition time is minimal. The difference this correction makes to the perfusion-weighted image can be seen in Figure 3.5.

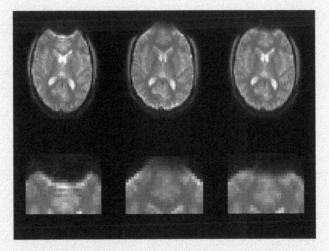

Figure 3.4: A slice from the calibration images: with AP phase encoding (left) and PA encoding (center). From these, a field map has been estimated and used to combine the two to create a corrected calibration image (right).

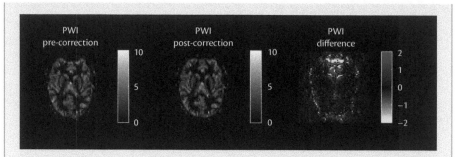

Figure 3.5: A slice from the perfusion-weighted image before (left) and after (center) distortion correction. The difference between the two (right) shows that the majority of the change occurs in the anterior region, as might be expected from the distortion seen in Figure 3.4.

On the primer website, you will find this dataset along with instructions on how to estimate the distortion correction from the calibration images and apply this approach to obtain both a corrected calibration image as well as corrected ASL difference data.

Another process that makes the data look distorted is seen in ASL data acquired using a 3D imaging readout. Blurring can be seen in one direction in the data, most commonly in the inferior–superior direction; this arises owing to increased T_2 decay of the signals during the longer readout period compared with 2D ASL data (see Section 2.3). If it is present, an inferior–superior blur can often be seen when looking at a sagittal or coronal view, its effect is not at all obvious from the normal axial slice; see Example Box 3.3. This is often reduced by altering the ASL sequence parameters and effectively breaking up (or segmenting) the acquisition as discussed in Section 2.3. It is, however, possible to account for the blurring in the 3D readout by using a "deblurring" method. Correction is achieved by a process that is essentially the same as "sharpening" a picture, but only applied in the through-slice direction.

Example Box 3.3: **Blurring in 3D GRASE ASL**

Figure 3.6 shows a fairly extreme example of the effect of blurring in a 3D GRASE acquisition. In this case, it was not a segmented acquisition, and so each volume was acquired in a single shot, which is no longer commonly done with 3D GRASE ASL. The blurring can be seen in the calibration image (top row), but is more obvious in the difference image (row 3), although it is only visible when viewing sagittal or coronal slices; the axial slice looks acceptably like a perfusion-weighted image. Deblurring has been applied to both images (rows 2 and 4) and can be seen to have reduced the effect, but also to have introduced noise, most obvious in the corrected difference image (row 4).

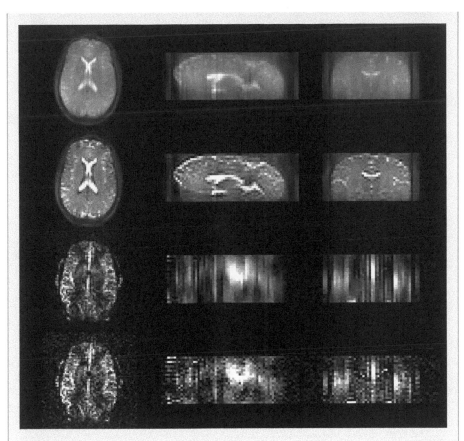

Figure 3.6: An example of ASL data acquired using 3D GRASE with only a single "shot" (not segmented), central slice for all three views. The top two rows are the original calibration image and the result after correction for blurring. The bottom two rows show pre- and post-deblurring for the ASL difference image (mean of 10 repeats).

3.3 Registration

As with many other MRI data, there is often a need to transform low-resolution ASL data from a subject into a different resolution and orientation. The most obvious example is the need to transform the images from a group of subjects into a common space, such as the MNI152 standard space for group analysis (see Chapter 8). The challenges posed by doing this for ASL data, with low resolution and low contrast, are shared with BOLD fMRI, and the processes for achieving acceptable registration are similar: namely, initial rigid registration of ASL data to a structural image coupled with the (usually non-linear) registration of the structural image to the standard space (or template). This process is illustrated in Figure 3.7, where a linear rigid-body

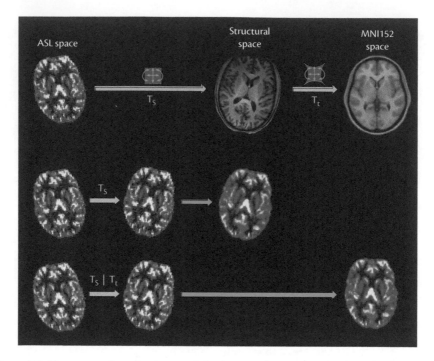

Figure 3.7: The process of transforming a perfusion image so that it is aligned with another brain image such as the T_1-weighted structural image in the same subject or a template such as the MNI152 standard brain. Registration is required to estimate the transformations T_s and T_t; these can be used to transform the image and interpolation can be used to match the voxel size to that of the target image.

registration has been used to estimate the transformation T_s needed to align the ASL data to a T_1-weighted structural image in the same subject. A second, non-linear, registration has been used to estimate the transformation T_t between the T_1-weighted structural image and a template, in this case the MNI152 standard brain. These transformations can then be applied along with interpolation to produce perfusion images that are aligned and have the same voxel size as either the structural or the template image. Further details on common approaches to registration of neuroimaging data can be found in the primer in this series "Introduction to Neuroimaging Analysis."

As with motion correction, background suppression does not assist in this registration process, and the calibration images are often a more useful basis for the first registration step (ensuring that any motion between the main ASL data and the calibration images is also corrected for). The ASL perfusion image often provides the best contrast between gray and white matter, owing to physiological differences between tissue types as well as partial volume effects (something that we will consider further in Chapter 6), and thus is often the best basis for registration, albeit a noisy one. A pragmatic solution, therefore is to use a preliminary registration between the calibration and structural images for initialization of that between the perfusion and structural images. This procedure is illustrated in Example Box 3.4.

Example Box 3.4: Transforming the perfusion image into structural space

Figure 3.8 shows the perfusion image from Chapter 1 once registration has been used to transform it to the same resolution as the T_1 structural image, shown alongside. In Figure 3.9, the perfusion image is shown overlaid on top of the structural image. From this, you can spot how the regions of highest perfusion correspond to regions of gray matter, either in the cortex or in deep gray matter structures.

On the primer website, you will find this dataset along with instructions on how to perform the registration between ASL data and a T_1 structural image, which then allows for the transformation of the final perfusion image into T_1 structural space.

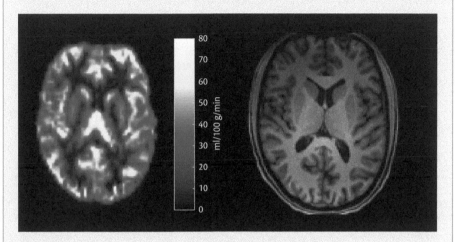

Figure 3.8: A slice through the perfusion image (left) once it has been transformed into the same space as the structural image alongside the structural image (right) at the same location.

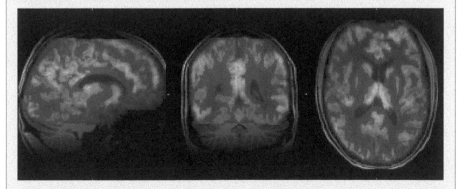

Figure 3.9: Views of the perfusion image (red–yellow) overlaid onto the structural image.

3.4 Spatial filtering

Since ASL data is inherently low-SNR, some degree of spatial filtering (smoothing) of the data can be helpful for visualization and also for group analysis, as is done with other neuroimaging data; see the primer in this series: "Introduction to Neuroimaging Analysis." For data acquired all at the same PLD, it does not matter whether the label–control data or the final perfusion image is subject to smoothing. However, data containing different PLDs (or label durations) should not be smoothed before model-fitting (see Section 4.7), since mixing different voxels with different ATTs could lead to poorer quality fitting and bias in the final perfusion estimates. A small (subvoxel) degree of smoothing, prior to model fitting, has some value, because this step can reduce the worst of the noise in the data and can lead to an overall better result in voxels where the non-linear model fitting otherwise failed to converge.

Standard spatial filtering involves setting a fixed spatial extent parameter, which neglects the fact that some areas of the volume may have more inherent smoothness than others or may exhibit different noise levels. A useful alternative is to let the data dictate the smoothing used, something that is offered by spatial priors in Bayesian model inversion, which we will meet in chapter 4. This is applied directly to the perfusion image (and not the data), as part of the model fitting, making it suitable for both single- and multi-PLD ASL.

SUMMARY

- Motion of the subject's head during acquisition is an issue for generating perfusion images and leads to artifacts in the label–control subtraction.
- Motion correction is generally recommended for ASL data, but cannot perfectly resolve subtraction artifacts, so inspection of the data to identify where these have occurred is important.
- Different readouts can lead to distortion of the images, some of which can be at least partially corrected for as part of the preprocessing, but might require the acquisition of additional data to estimate the extent of the effect; for example, a field map may be required.
- Registration of the perfusion map to a structural image is often required. The perfusion image provides the best gray–white matter contrast for registration to the structural image, but may be noisy. First registering the calibration image to the structural image is often a good way to provide an initial guess of the transformation, which can be improved upon using the perfusion image.
- Spatial smoothing can be beneficial, especially for visualization, but some quantification method might offer their own adaptive spatial smoothing that may be preferable if the data is to be used for further analysis, such as group analysis.

FURTHER READING

■ Chappell, M. and Jenkinson, M. (2017). *Introduction to Neuroimaging Analysis* (Oxford Neuroimaging Primers). Oxford University Press.
  ■ *The introductory primer to this series provides more details on the motivation and common approaches for the preprocessing methods discussed in this chapter.*

■ Shirzadi, Z., Crane, D. E., Robertson, A. D., Maralani, P. J., Aviv, R. I., Chappell, M. A., et al. (2015). Automated removal of spurious intermediate cerebral blood flow volumes improves image quality among older patients: A clinical arterial spin labeling investigation. *Journal of Magnetic Resonance Imaging*, 42(5), 1377–1385.
  ■ *This is an example of a work in which motion correction has been combined with an automated process to reject individual volumes from the ASL time series to achieve a more robust perfusion image.*

■ Madai, V. I., Martin, S. Z., Samson Himmelstjerna, F. C., Herzig, C. X., Mutke, M. A., Wood, C. N., et al. (2016). Correction for susceptibility distortions increases the performance of arterial spin labeling in patients with cerebrovascular disease. *Journal of Neuroimaging*, 26(4), 436–444.
  ■ *This is an example where susceptibility distortion correction was evaluated within the context of an ASL-based study.*

■ Chappell, M. A., Groves, A. R., Macintosh, B. J., Donahue, M. J., Jezzard, P. & Woolrich, M. W. (2011). Partial volume correction of multiple inversion time arterial spin labeling MRI data. *Magnetic Resonance in Medicine*, 65(4), 1173–1183.
  ■ *In this work, the authors used a "deblurring" approach to correct for through-plane blurring-based distortion of GRASE ASL data.*

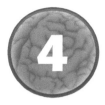

Kinetic Modeling

The label–control difference signal measured in an ASL experiment can be described according to tracer kinetics, where we treat the labeled blood-water as a tracer whose "concentration," of hydrogen nuclei with inverted magnetization (see Chapter 2), gives rise to the measured signal. The reason that we need a tracer kinetic model is that we want to relate the signal we measure at the PLD to the amount of labeled blood-water that has been delivered. As we saw in Chapter 1, the end result of the kinetic model is a formula that allows us to convert from signal value to absolute perfusion (in ml/100 g/min), as long as we also have a measure of the magnetization of arterial blood to calibrate our signal—something that we will discuss in Chapter 5. In this chapter, we are going to construct a simple model of the labeled blood-water tracer so that you can understand the assumptions that go into that formula and thus also its limitations. We will then consider various extensions and modifications to the model that we might use to correct for various artifacts or if we want to extract other hemodynamic information, e.g., ATT when using multi-PLD ASL.

We know that labeled blood-water is generated in the neck and delivered to the tissue by the vasculature. Once it reaches the voxel, it remains there for some time, determined by how long it takes either for the labeled water to leave the voxel again or for the label to decay owing to T_1 relaxation. The essential components of our kinetic model are descriptions of tracer delivery and tracer removal; in tracer kinetics, these are often called the *arterial input function* and the *residue function*.

The *arterial input function* (AIF) describes the time course of delivery of the labeled blood-water to the part of the brain being imaged. It allows us to account for the "shape" of the bolus of tracer that has been created. For example, we use it to account for the label duration and thus the total amount of labeled-blood water that we have created, as well as the time taken for the labeled blood to reach the tissue.

The *residue function* describes what proportion of the labeled blood-water that arrived in the voxel at a particular point in time still remains sometime later. This means that the residue function must equal one at time equal to zero, since on arrival the contrast has not yet had time to leave. The residue function cannot increase, since that would require the creation of new labeled blood-water within the voxel. Owing to the magnetization decay process, labeled blood-water decays away over time once it has arrived, and thus the residue function will decrease with time.

We can notionally break up the bolus of labeled blood-water, i.e., the arterial input function, into lots of small pieces that arrive sequentially. The residue function tells us what happens to each piece and how much we will have left some time later. If we want to know how much labeled water we have in the voxel, and thus the signal we will measure, we can then combine the arterial input function with the residue function, summing up all the contributions from the "pieces" of the bolus of labeled blood-water that have been delivered. This process is illustrated in Figure 4.1. The final thing we need to account for is the rate at which labeled blood-water is delivered to the voxel, i.e., the perfusion. Since the AIF captures the concentration of the tracer in the blood, the perfusion is simply a multiplier on the final expression for the ASL signal we measure in the voxel. Mathematically, we are performing the convolution of the two functions and then multiplication with the perfusion, which is described in Box 4.1.

Box 4.1: The general tracer kinetic model

Formally, classic tracer kinetics relates the concentration $C(t)$ of a contrast agent in a region to the rate of delivery, i.e., the perfusion f, by

$$C(t) = f \cdot a(t) \otimes r(t) = f \int_0^t a(\xi) r(t - \xi) \, d\xi$$

where

    $a(t)$ is the arterial input function,
    $r(t)$ is the residue function, and
    $\otimes$ signifies convolution, as defined by the integral on the right-hand side of the
    equation, where ξ is a "dummy" variable.

By definition, $r(0) = 1$ and $r(t + \delta t) \leq r(t)$ for any positive time increment δt. This captures the requirement that the residue function tells us about what happens to the tracer once it has arrived: namely, it is all present initially (time since arrival equals zero) and it can only remain or be lost (leave the region or decay), not created, although more can be delivered via $a(t)$.

4.1 The simplest ASL kinetic model

We will start out with the simplest model possible, which is the same one we used in Chapter 1, but we will consider in more detail how the kinetic model is formed and also how this applies to both pcASL and pASL labeling.

4.1.1 Arterial input function (AIF)

The ASL contrast is generated by radiofrequency inversion either applied for a brief time over a region as in pulsed labeling or applied to blood flowing through a plane for a set period of time, as in (pseudo-)continuous labeling. Both methods, in the ideal case, create a rectangular profile of labeled blood-water. This function is a box-car (top-hat) shape at the site of labeling, with the

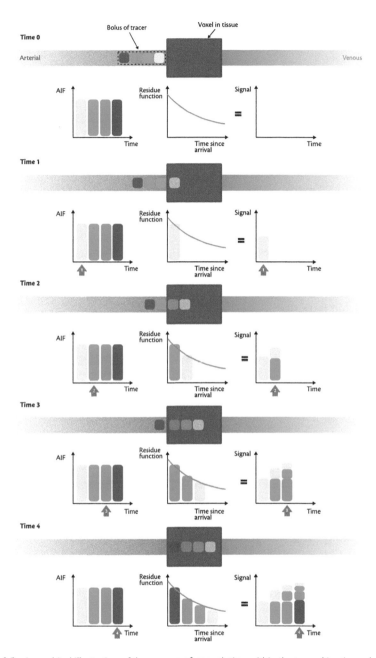

Figure 4.1: A graphical illustration of the process of convolution within the tracer kinetic model. As time progresses, more of the bolus of tracer (this would be the labeled blood-water in an ASL experiment) arrives in the region of interest (the red box representing a voxel in the tissue); this delivery is described by the arterial input function (AIF). The longer the tracer remains in the tissue, the more it decays (like the T_1 decay of the label in ASL); this is described by the residue function. The measured signal is the sum of all the contributions from the tracer that has been delivered in whatever state of decay it is. Thus, in this case, the signal increases over time, with tracer that was delivered at earlier times contributing progressively less and less to the total signal the longer it remains in the voxel.

duration of the function set by the label duration for the pcASL case or the size of the labeling region and speed of blood flow through it for the pASL case, as discussed in Section 2.1.

At the same time, the label is decaying at a rate determined by the T_1 value. The effect will be different for the two labeling schemes: for pASL, we label a spatially defined region of blood all at once—this means that the tail end of the bolus will take longer to reach the voxel and thus will have decayed more compared with the leading edge by the time it reaches the voxel; for pcASL, we label blood as it passes through a plane so the time between inversion and arrival at the voxel is fixed and the whole bolus will experience the same amount of label decay. Figure 4.2(a) plots the pASL and pcASL arterial input functions using the recommended labeling parameters from the consensus paper (with QUIPSS II pulses for pASL to limit the label duration), mathematical expressions can be found in Box 4.2. Notice that the area under the curve of the pASL function is smaller than that of the pcASL function, owing to the shorter label duration that can be achieved and the T_1 decay that reduces the intensity over time. This is significant, since it represents the total amount of label that we can possibly deliver to the voxel for a given perfusion. The difference between the two AIFs is one of the major motivations for (p)cASL labeling, as with a longer label duration and less pronounced T_1 decay more labeled water can be delivered and a bigger signal achieved.

4.1.2 Residue function

Since ASL is based on labeling blood-water, the residue function must describe what happens to that water once it arrives in the voxel. We will assume that in the voxel the label has made it as far as the capillary bed—it is in the "tissue." According to the definition that we have given, the residue function needs to describe how much remains some time after arrival. There are two routes by which labeled water might "leave": by passing through capillaries and out the venous side, or by magnetization decay. In our simplest model, we will assume that no label physically leaves the voxel, it simply "stays and decays." This is based on the argument that there is not enough time for the label to pass through the capillary bed and exit the voxel before T_1 decay has effectively removed most of it. This residue function is shown in Figure 4.2(b): it is a simple exponential decay function governed by T_1, in this case the T_1 of blood at 3 T as recommended by the consensus paper; the equation for this function is given in Box 4.2.

4.1.3 Kinetic model

The final kinetic model is generated by performing the convolution of the two functions; the equations that result can be found in Box 4.2. This gives a mathematical description of the signal in the label–control difference image that we would expect to observe at any point in time after labeling and thus allows us to relate measured signal to perfusion. Example time series for pASL and pcASL are shown in Figure 4.2(c) using the recommended values from the consensus paper and the same value of perfusion in both cases. For both labeling schemes, the recommended PLD or TI is shown—the value for pASL being shorter than for pcASL because of the shorter label duration that can be achieved by labeling a region of the neck (see Section 2.1). This compensates somewhat for the lower total "concentration" of label that can be achieved with pASL. It might seem strange how late the recommended PLD or TI is compared with the maximum signal intensity; this has to do with variation in the time it takes for the labeled blood-water to arrive in the voxel, something we will consider in Box 4.4, once we have extended our model.

Box 4.2: The simplest ASL kinetic model equations

Arterial input function

We can describe the AIF mathematically as

$$a(t) = \begin{cases} 0 & t < 0 \\ 2M_{0a}e^{-t/T_{1b}} & \text{(pASL)} \quad 0 \leq t < \tau \\ 2M_{0a} & \text{(pcASL)} \\ 0 & t \geq \tau \end{cases}$$

where

M_{0a} is the magnetization of the arterial blood when in the labeling region,
T_{1b} is the T1 of the arterial blood, and
τ is the label duration.

Notice that the magnetization of the arterial blood appears here as the amplitude of the function. This represents the total magnetization we have available to us from which we can create our label. But notice also the factor of two that appears because we are labeling using inversion, which reverses the direction of the magnetization—the hydrogen nuclei go from having a magnetization of $+M_{0a}$ to $-M_{0a}$, a difference of $2M_{0a}$. Because we are working with the label–control subtraction signal (and we always calculate control minus label), we do not have to worry about the sign change and can treat the AIF as having a magnitude of $2M_{0a}$. These functions are those plotted in Figure 4.2(a) with $M_{0a} = 1$.

Residue function

Mathematically, our simple residue function is

$$R(t) = e^{-t/T_1}$$

where T_1 is that of the labeled water when it is in the voxel. Note that the residue function is a property of the tissue in the voxel and therefore does not depend upon how we do the labeling.

Kinetic model

We can write down (by performing the convolution) the appropriate model for the difference in magnetization between label and control conditions for pcASL acquisitions as

$$\Delta M(t) = 0 \qquad t < 0$$
$$2M_{0a}fT_{1b}\left(1 - e^{-t/T_{1b}}\right) \qquad 0 \leq t < \tau$$
$$2M_{0a}fT_{1b}e^{-t/T_{1b}}\left(e^{\tau/T_{1b}} - 1\right) \qquad \tau \leq t$$

The same can be done for pASL:

$$\Delta M(t) = 0 \qquad t < 0$$
$$2M_{0a}fe^{-t/T_{1b}}t \qquad 0 \leq t < \tau$$
$$2M_{0a}fe^{-t/T_{1b}}\tau \qquad \tau \leq t$$

These are plotted in Figure 4.2(c) with $M_{0a} \cdot f = 1$.

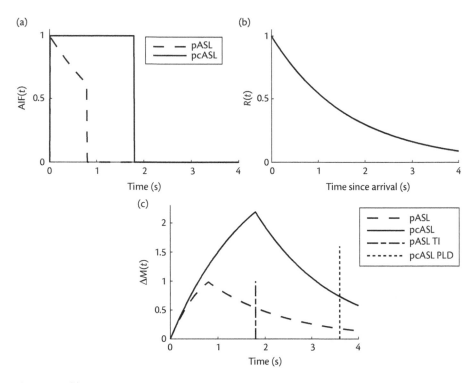

Figure 4.2: (a) Time series plot of the arterial input function for pcASL and pASL using the recommendations in the consensus paper (a bolus duration of 1.8 s for pcASL and 0.8 s for pASL) and assuming T_1 decay with time constant of 1.65 s. (b) Time series plot of the residue function that captures the decay of the labeled blood-water after arrival in the voxel with a T_1 time constant of 1.65 s. (c) Time series plot of the kinetic model of labeled-blood water in a voxel based on the simple model for both pcASL and pASL using the recommended parameters in the consensus paper and showing the recommended PLD or TI at which measurement would occur.

4.2 The standard model

The simplest kinetic model for ASL can be used for quantification of perfusion from ASL data and is the recommended solution for single-PLD data according to the consensus paper. However, it is more common in the literature on ASL kinetics to come across the "standard" model.

4.2.1 Arterial input function

The standard model makes the same assumptions about the arterial input function as we did for the simple model. However, since the labeling will have been performed remotely from the imaging region, there will be a delay in the arrival of the label at the voxel depending upon the length of the path it takes through the vasculature and speed of flow in the vessels. Since the AIF describes the label that actually arrives at the voxel, it will be a shifted version of the function at the labeling site, with the shift being equal to the *arterial transit time* (ATT), which is sometimes called the arterial arrival time or bolus arrival time. This will, in turn, affect how much the labeled blood-water has decayed by the time we observe it. For pcASL, in which the blood is labeled as it passes through a plane, all blood takes the same time to reach the voxel and thus will have all experienced the same T_1 decay—related to the ATT for the voxel. For pASL, the label will have also decayed in transit, but, as in the simple model, the trailing edge will have decayed more since it will have taken longer to arrive. These effects are illustrated in the plots in Figure 4.3, where a range of different ATTs are shown; the modified equations for the AIF with ATT are given in Box 4.3.

4.2.2 Residue function

For the residue function, we can be a little more precise about what happens to the label when it arrives in the voxel. We will now separately describe the two processes by which the label "leaves," as also described mathematically in Box 4.3.

In the first process, the label exits the voxel by leaving the capillary bed on the venous side: the key assumption in the standard model is that water is freely diffusible across the capillary membrane. Thus, the labeled water rapidly exchanges between the capillary blood and the surrounding tissue, appearing both in the extracellular extravascular space and within the cells. This leads to the "well-mixed" assumption, whereby we assume that the concentrations of the label in capillary blood and tissue reach equilibrium sufficiently rapidly that the voxel can be

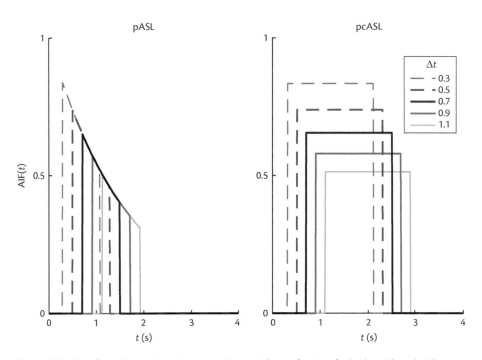

Figure 4.3: The effect of arterial transit time on the arterial input function for both pcASL and pASL.

treated as a well-mixed volume of water. This means that the concentration at the venous end of the capillary bed will simply equal that of the label distributed throughout the voxel. The rate of removal on the venous end will equal that of delivery, namely, the perfusion. A further refinement is to take into account that the concentration of water in blood differs from that in tissue—the two being related by the partition coefficient (discussed in more detail in Chapter 5).

The second process is the relaxation of the label with T_1 once it has arrived in the voxel. Since the tissue volume far exceeds that of the capillaries, it is reasonable to assume that the majority of the labeled water is within the tissue and thus decays with the T_1 of the tissue, which will be shorter than that of the blood we used for the AIF.

In practice, the venous outflow in the standard model is insignificant, and so effectively the model is like the simple model and assumes all the label arrives in the tissue and stays there, decaying with T_1.

4.2.3 Kinetic model

Figure 4.4 shows examples of the time series for the kinetic model for both pASL and pcASL as the key parameters, namely, ATT, label duration, and T_1 of tissue, are varied, but with perfusion kept at the same value. The equations for this model can be found in Box 4.3. Notice that at the recommended PLD (or TI), both methods are relatively insensitive to ATT, as long as it does not exceed a particularly long time, which is dependent on the choice of acquisition parameters. Sensitivity to label duration means that it is important that the actual label duration be known for the purposes of quantification of perfusion. Both methods are relatively insensitive to T_1 (a comparatively large range has been used here for visualization purposes, compared with what might be expected in vivo). Having now got a description of the general kinetic model for the ASL tracer we can now use this to help with the choice of a good PLD for acquisition in Box 4.4.

If we have multi-PLD (or multi-TI) data, we can use this model (or even the simple model from Section 4.1) to estimate both perfusion and ATT using methods that we will discuss in Section 4.7—something that is illustrated in Example Box 4.1.

Box 4.3: The standard ASL kinetic model equations

Arterial input function

The AIFs including ATT, Δt, are given by

$$a(t) = \begin{cases} 0 & t < \Delta t \\ 2M_{0a}e^{-(t-\Delta t)/T_{1b}} & \text{(pASL)} \quad \Delta t \leq t < \tau + \Delta t \\ 2M_{0a}e^{-\Delta t/T_{1b}} & \text{(pcASL)} \\ 0 & \tau + \Delta t \leq t \end{cases}$$

These are plotted in Figure 4.3 with $M_{0a} = 1$.

Residue function

We can write the residue function as the product of two terms:

$$R(t) = r(t)m(t)$$

with

$r(t) = e^{-t \cdot f/\lambda}$ capturing the outflow effect that depends on the partition coefficient λ, and $m(t) = e^{-t/T_1}$ capturing the magnetization decay with the T_1 of the tissue in the voxel.

The only difference then from the simple model is the $r(t)$ term, and with a "normal" perfusion (in gray matter) of 60 ml/100 g/min (which is 0.01 s^{-1}) and a λ of 0.9, this decay, with a time constant of the order of 100 s, is slow compared with T_1, which is typically of the order of a few seconds.

Kinetic model

We can write down (by performing the convolution) the equations for the difference in magnetization between label and control conditions for pcASL acquisitions as

$$\Delta M(t) = \begin{cases} 0 & t < \Delta t \\ 2M_{0a}fT_{1app}e^{-\Delta t/T_{1b}}\left(1-e^{-(t-\Delta t)/T_{1app}}\right) & \Delta t \le t < \Delta t + \tau \\ 2M_{0a}fT_{1app}e^{-\Delta t/T_{1b}}e^{-(t-\Delta t-\tau)/T_{1app}}\left(1-e^{-\tau/T_{1app}}\right) & \Delta t + \tau \le t \end{cases}$$

where $1/T_{1app} = 1/T_1 + f/\lambda$.

The same can be done for pASL:

$$\Delta M(t) = 0 \qquad\qquad\qquad\qquad t < \Delta t$$
$$2M_{0a}fT_{1r}e^{-t/T_{1app}}\left(e^{t/T_{1r}} - e^{\Delta t/T_{1r}}\right) \qquad \Delta t \le t < \Delta t + \tau$$
$$2M_{0a}fT_{1r}e^{-t/T_{1app}}\left(e^{(\Delta t+\tau)/T_{1r}} - e^{\Delta t/T_{1r}}\right) \qquad \Delta t + \tau \le t$$

where $1/T_{1r} = 1/T_{1app} - 1/T_{1b}$.

These are plotted in Figure 4.4 with $M_{0a} \cdot f = 1$.

Box 4.4: Choosing a PLD to be insensitive to ATT

As discussed in Chapters 1 and 2, sensitivity to ATT is an important confound for accurate perfusion measurement for single PLD ASL. The approach recommended by the consensus paper is to choose a PLD such that the signal is largely insensitive to ATT, on the falling part of the kinetic curve. Their recommendations for pASL and the choice of TI follow a similar logic. These recommended measurement times are shown in Figure 4.4, which illustrates that there are a range of ATT values for which the measurement will be largely insensitive to ATT, but there is a limit. For pcASL, this comes when the ATT exceeds the PLD, and with the consensus paper recommendations this yields ATTs beyond 1.8 s. This should be a fairly safe choice in many subjects, but could be problematic in elderly subjects and especially in some pathologies such as steno-occlusive disease, where slower blood flow rates lead to prolonged ATT. For example, in elderly subjects, the consensus paper recommends a PLD of 2 s.

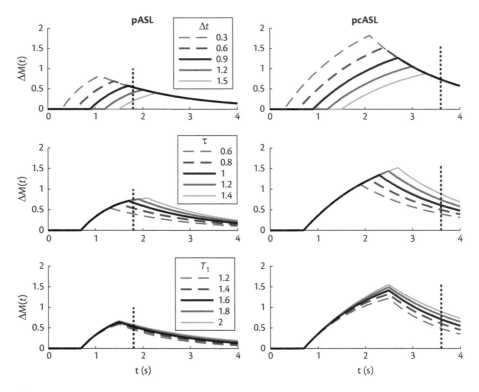

Figure 4.4: Variation in the ASL signal, at a voxel in the brain, with respect to changes in ATT, T_1, and bolus duration, for both pcASL and pASL. The recommended measurement times (PLD or TI) for both pcASL and pASL are shown based on the consensus paper. In practice the ATT, Δt, achieved by pcASL labeling is often longer than via pASL, although a value of 0.7 s has been used here for visualisation, excepted where otherwise indicated.

Example Box 4.1: Multi-PLD pcASL

For the subject we first met in Chapter 1, we also have a set of multi-PLD pcASL data that has been analyzed using model fitting. This data has all the same parameters as that of the set in Chapter 1, except a shorter label duration of 1.4 s and six different PLDs, with each repeated eight times: 0.25, 0.5, 0.75, 1.0, 1.25, 1.5 s. The difference images at each PLD (after averaging over the repeated measurements) are shown in Figure 4.5. Notice that the voxel intensities typically start high and decrease at later PLDs because we are primarily sampling the tail of the kinetic curve, but in posterior regions labeled blood water has not yet arrived at the shortest PLD and only appears in later PLDs.

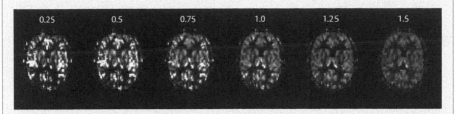

Figure 4.5: The label–control difference images at different PLD values (in seconds), after averaging over the repeated measurements of each PLD.

Figure 4.6 shows the central slice of the perfusion image from this multi-PLD data alongside that from the single-PLD data. The overall spatial distribution is very similar between the two cases, although the perfusion estimated from the single PLD is slightly higher, corresponding to the implicit assumption that ATT is zero in the quantification for single PLD given in Box 1.3. Also shown is the ATT map, estimated using the multiple PLDs; this is noisier than the perfusion image, particularly in regions of low perfusion (i.e., the white matter). The more prolonged ATT in the posterior of the brain is quite typical and matches with the later arrival of labeled blood-water in these regions in Figure 4.5.

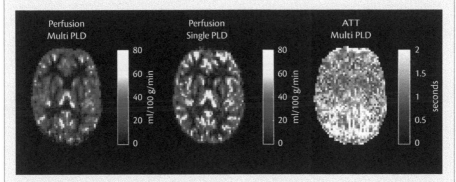

Figure 4.6: The central slice of the perfusion image from the multi-PLD pcASL data (left) alongside the perfusion image in the same subject acquired with a single PLD (center). The multi-PLD data also provides a map of ATT (right).

On the primer website, you will find the data used in this example, along with instructions on how to compute the perfusion and ATT maps shown here.

4.3 Signal components: arterial signal contamination

We have, up to this point, assumed that the only signal we observe in the ASL difference image arises from labeled blood-water delivered to the tissue. Because it takes some time for the blood to pass through the vasculature on its way to the tissue, we might also observe signal arising from labeled blood-water still in the arteries on its way to tissue as we saw in Section 2.7. As per the definition in Chapter 1, this signal is not reflective of perfusion, since the blood-water giving rise to the signal is responsible for delivery to tissue downstream from the artery. The recommended PLD values in the consensus paper were chosen to try to reduce this effect by leaving plenty of time for labeled blood to reach the tissue, having already passed through the arteries. Alternatively, flow suppression (see Section 2.7) can be used to suppress the contribution from hydrogen nuclei moving in the blood based on the velocity of their motion and thus aims to remove this signal.

An alternative, which is possible when the data has multiple PLDs, is to include this effect as a separate component within the model—the *arterial signal component*, sometimes called the macrovascular signal component, as it is presumed to arise from the larger vessels in the vasculature but might include some smaller vessels too (see also Box 4.7).

4.3.1 Arterial signal component

We can model the arterial signal for the standard model by using the arterial input function (see Box 4.5), since when we observe an arterial signal what we are observing is the signal from labeled blood-water in the arteries that is passing through on its way to tissue elsewhere. The scaling of the signal will be related to the magnetization of the arterial blood—the concentration of the tracer—and the amount of arterial blood contained within the voxel. Thus, the arterial component gives rise to a new parameter, the *arterial cerebral blood volume* (aCBV). This should not be confused with the blood volume metrics provided by other perfusion imaging methods, which capture the total volume of blood within the voxel, since for the arterial component it is only the *arterial* blood that contributes; for more on this, see Box 4.6.

Box 4.5: Arterial component model

The equation for the arterial component is very similar to that for the AIF, since essentially that is what is being observed, albeit in the artery before it arrives at the tissue:

$$A(t) = \begin{cases} 0 & & t < \Delta t_a \\ 2M_{0a} \cdot aCBV \cdot e^{-(t-\Delta t)/T_{1b}} & \text{(pASL)} & \Delta t_a \leq t < \tau + \Delta t_a \\ 2M_{0a} \cdot aCBV \cdot e^{-\Delta t/T_{1b}} & \text{(pcASL)} & \\ 0 & & \tau + \Delta t_a \leq t \end{cases}$$

where

aCBV is the arterial cerebral blood volume and

Δt_a is the first arrival of the labeled blood-water in the artery within the voxel, sometimes called the bolus arrival time (BAT), although this term has also been used to describe the first arrival in the tissue (i.e., the ATT) in some earlier literature.

Strictly speaking, this model only holds as long as the labeled blood passes sufficiently rapidly through the voxel that it does not dwell for long in the voxel and that there is negligible exchange of labeled water between the blood in the artery and the surrounding tissue. This will generally be true for larger arteries, where the flow speed will be of the order of 10 cm/s for voxels of size of the order of 5 mm.

Box 4.6: Can ASL measure cerebral blood volume?

As noted in Chapter 1, the way in which ASL measures perfusion is different to other MR perfusion imaging modalities. If you are already familiar with other perfusion imaging methods, such as dynamic susceptibility contrast (DSC) perfusion-weighted MRI, you might wonder whether you can get similar measures, such as the cerebral blood volume, from ASL. Despite ASL being a tracer-based method, that fact that it uses water as a tracer means that we do not necessarily get the same measures of hemodynamics. For example, in DSC MRI, the gadolinium-based tracer remains intravascular in the brain (except in certain pathologies), and this makes it possible to derive a measure of blood volume within any given voxel from the data. Since the ASL tracer largely leaves the vasculature, getting a classic measure of blood volume from all the different parts of the vasculature within the voxel will not be possible. This means that ASL cannot measure the "mean transit time," a common metric in other perfusion imaging methods, which is the average time it takes the tracer to transit the vasculature within the voxel. This should not be confused with the ATT, which measures time taken before arriving in the voxel through the arterial vasculature. As we have seen from considering the macrovascular signal arising from ASL-labeled blood-water still within the arteries, we can get a measure of arterial blood volume from ASL, but this measure is strictly limited to the large arteries.

Estimation of this signal component can be achieved from multi-PLD data using model fitting (see Section 4.7), which is illustrated in Figure 4.7 and is explored in Example Box 4.2. Sequences that include a mixture of acquisitions with and without flow suppression offer particular benefits for extracting the arterial signal and information about the AIF; see Box 4.13.

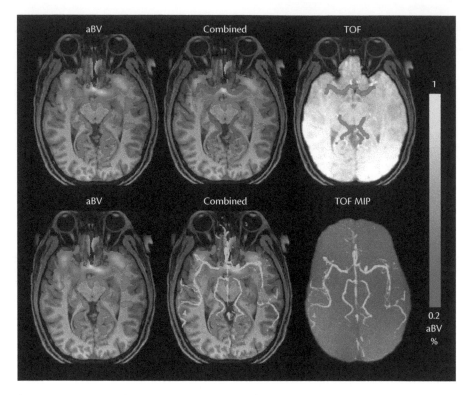

Figure 4.7: An example of aCBV estimated from ASL data (in this case a multi-TI pASL variant) shown overlaid on the structural image on the left and in the center, with an angiographic image (the time-of-flight image in the same slice in the top row and the maximum-intensity projection through the whole brain in the bottom row) in the same subject, showing the location of major arteries on the right and overlaid on the other images in the center. Major vascular structures can be seen in both the ASL estimates and the more commonly used angiographic readout, providing evidence that an arterial signal can be extracted from ASL data.

Reproduced with permission from Chappell, M. A., MacIntosh, B. J., Donahue, M. J., Günther, M., Jezzard, P., & Woolrich, M. W., 'Separation of macrovascular signal in multi-inversion time arterial spin labelling MRI', *Magnetic Resonance in Medicine*, Volume 63, Issue 5, pp. 1357–1365, DOI: 10.1002/mrm.22320, Copyright © 2010 Wiley-Liss, Inc.

Example Box 4.2: **Macrovascular contamination in multi-PLD pcASL**

Figure 4.8 shows the multi-PLD pcASL data from Figure 4.6 when it has been analyzed using an additional arterial component. Three slices are shown that are more inferior to the one shown in Example Box 4.1 This is where most of the arterial contamination is expected for two reasons: first, larger arteries are found toward the base of the brain; second, the 2D readout means that more-superior slices have longer PLD and thus are less likely to be contaminated by arterial signal. The aCBV map shows evidence of common vascular structures such as the circle of Willis in the most inferior slices shown here (top row), as well as the posterior cerebral arteries (middle row) and branches of the middle cerebral artery (bottom row).

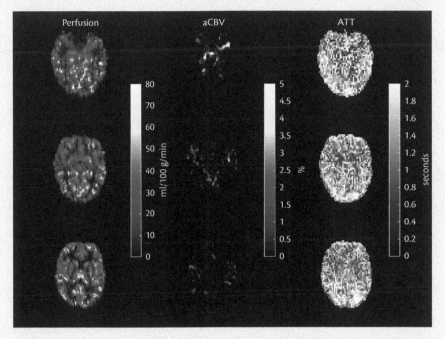

Figure 4.8: Three slices from the multi-PLD pcASL dataset analyzed with both tissue and arterial components, giving rise to a perfusion image (left) along with maps of arterial cerebral blood volume (center) and ATT (right). These are more-inferior brain slices compared with those in Figure 4.6.

On the primer website, you will find the data used in this example, along with instructions on how to compute the perfusion, aCBV and ATT maps shown here.

4.3.2 Other signal components

Labeled blood-water that is still in the major arteries is the main source of signal that cannot be explained by the tissue model in ASL images, although it is less clear what we should make of vessels that lie in the range between arteries and capillaries; see Box 4.7. Under normal physiological conditions, the contribution of labeled blood in the venous vasculature is liable to be minimal and not observable. The standard model assumes that there is some venous outflow of label from the well-mixed tissue compartment. However, the contribution is very small—of the order of 1% of the ASL difference signal for a perfusion of 60 ml/100g/min (0.01 s^{-1}). In practice, any venous signal would not be observed until the labeled water had traversed the capillary bed (the standard model has a zero transit time under the well-mixed assumption), so the signal would be reduced even further by T_1 decay during transit. The only time this might not be true is in pathologies, such as arteriovenous malformation, where blood shunts directly from arterial to venous circulation.

> **Box 4.7: ASL signals from other parts of the vasculature**
>
> For the purpose of modeling so far, we have considered two extremes:
>
> > *microvasculature* (tissue), where label accumulates rapidly owing to fast exchange, and
> > *macrovasculature* (arteries), where label passes through rapidly and there is negligible
> > exchange.
>
> There is potential for signal to arise from smaller arteries and also arterioles, where
> the exchange of labeled water might still be small compared with that in the capillary
> bed, but where the speed of flow is such that blood dwells for some time within the
> voxel. It is likely that it would be hard to reliably distinguish this condition from that
> of the tissue signal, and it is unlikely to be beneficial to do so, since this will occur
> sufficiently close to the "tissue" that it still reasonably contributes to our measure of
> perfusion. However, we note here that we could model this effect by the convolution
> of the arterial input function with a box residue function with a duration equal to the
> "pre-capillary" dwell time.

4.4 Arterial input functions: modeling dispersion

The assumed form of the arterial function in the standard model reflects the way in which the
label is created. It is largely reasonable to assume that in the inversion region a well-defined
bolus of labeled blood is created, particularly for pcASL, where labeling occurs as blood passes
through a labeling plane. However, the labeled blood then has to pass through the vasculature
to reach the brain. The process of transit through progressively narrower vessels, flow in the
branching structure of the vasculature, and cardiac pulsation, will smooth the profile of the
idealized AIF, a process collectively termed *dispersion*.

A number of parameterized models exist to describe this process, of which the simplest
and also most successful for data analysis has been the *vascular transport function* (VTF) or
dispersion kernel; see Box 4.8. The VTF is a function that describes how severe the dispersion is. The VTF captures how a unit of tracer "spreads out" as it travels along the vasculature, and thus a broader VTF implies more dispersion. Overall, the effect of dispersion
is to "round off" the edges of the AIF, as is shown in Figure 4.9 for two popular VTFs for a
range of severity of dispersion. When applied using the sampling rates and typical SNR of
ASL data, it is difficult to distinguish between these different models in practice, even when
specifically observing the arterial signal. Thus, while dispersion can have an impact on the
estimated perfusion values, in practice it is often not important precisely which model is
chosen to describe the dispersion. However, the choice of model will affect what values
we get for ATT, and it has implications for the interpretation of this parameter, as discussed
in Box 4.9.

Box 4.8: **The vascular transport function model of dispersion**

Under the vascular transport function model, the dispersed AIF is given as

$$a'(t) = a(t) \otimes VTF(t)$$

where

$a'(t)$ is the dispersed AIF and

$VTF(t)$ is the vascular transport function.

The area under the curve for the VTF must be unity, since dispersion neither destroys nor creates label.

Two popular VTFs are the Gaussian and gamma functions, based on the respective probability distributions of the same names. The Gaussian VTF has a single dispersion parameter σ, whereas the gamma VTF has two degrees of freedom, with one version capturing these in two parameters: p, the "time to peak," and s, the "sharpness." It is variations of σ and s that are shown in Figure 4.9. Notice that the Gaussian function, being symmetric about zero, spreads the AIF in both directions along the time axis; in extreme cases, this can lead to labeled blood-water theoretically arriving before it is created.

Alternative models that have been proposed include the adoption of a gamma variate function, as has been used as the AIF in other perfusion modalities. This model, however, does not reconcile well with the idealized box-shaped bolus of the label created by ASL. Models have also been derived that more explicitly aim to model the effects of the flow profile in the arteries and the processes of mass transport. On the whole, these tend to be less useful for data analysis.

Box 4.9: **What is the arterial transit time when dispersion is present?**

For the non-dispersed AIF, the concept of the ATT was pretty obvious—it was associated with the sharp rise in the AIF due to the first arrival of labeled blood-water in the voxel. This then corresponds to the point where the ASL signal, described by the kinetic curve, starts to rise. We can adopt a similar definition when dispersion is present, but the interpretation of ATT and especially the comparison between analysis that corrects for dispersion and one without correction can become a little more complex. With dispersion, the first arrival of labeled blood-water in the voxel can be more subtle, as the leading edge of the bolus has been spread out in the flow. This is most obvious with the Gaussian VTF model in Figure 4.9: it is very hard to define where the curve starts to rise (and in some cases that point is clearly at $t < 0$, before the label has even been created). However, under this model, we reach 50% of the maximum signal at the same time as the ATT under the non-dispersed model. The effect is both similar and different for the gamma VTF model in Figure 4.9: again dispersion smears out the initial arrival of the bolus, making the rise gentler, but the time at which we reach a given fraction of the maximum signal now gets later with more dispersion. These effects ultimately manifest in the kinetic curve for the signal arising from the tissue in the voxel, making the initial rise of the curve gentler than in the standard model.

Commonly, we analyze ASL data using the standard model—without dispersion—whereas the data will arise from a bolus of labeled blood-water that will have experienced some dispersion. Because the standard model does not account for the gentle initial rise caused by dispersion, the ATT will most likely be estimated later than the very first arrival of labeled blood-water in the voxel, but will be associated with a point where a substantial fraction has arrived, making it somewhat sensitive to the amount of dispersion that has occurred. Thus, ATT is still a measure of the transit of blood through the vasculature to get to a region of the brain, but it is not the "first" arrival and may partially reflect other processes that happen to the blood on the way that give rise to dispersion. Thus, in a diseased population, ATT may no longer be due only to slowing blood flow, but also to dispersion (with the added possibility that slower flow could also lead to greater dispersion). Finally, given the differences in models of dispersion, an ATT estimated using a model of dispersion will not agree with the ATT from the standard model by definition, but neither will it agree with another model of dispersion.

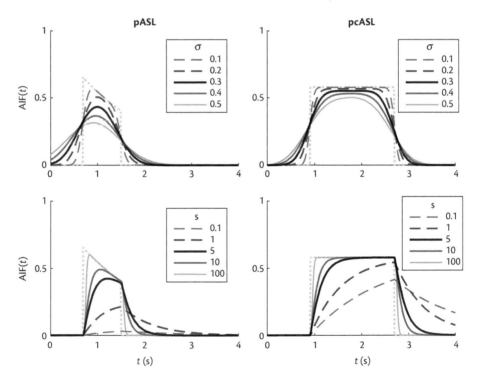

Figure 4.9: Examples of the effect of dispersion as modeled by a vascular transport function on pcASL and pASL arterial input functions for a Gaussian VTF (top) and a gamma VTF (bottom).

4.5 Residue functions: modeling restricted exchange

The assumption of the standard model was that labeled blood-water arrives into a well-mixed compartment. What this implies is that once the label arrives in the voxel, it immediately transfers out of the vessel, where it is evenly distributed across the volume. In reality, blood arrives into the voxel first in the capillaries, or even in arterioles. During its passage, there is opportunity for the labeled water to exchange out of the vessels, but it will not all do so instantaneously but progressively the further it travels through the voxel, and this will depend upon the rate of exchange of water between blood and tissue. It is reasonable to believe that the label exchanges quite easily between the blood and the extravascular space, since water is know to cross cell membranes fairly freely. However, there may be some delay during which the label is decaying with the T_1 of blood, before it enters the tissue and decays with the T_1 of tissue. Diseases that affect the transfer of substances across the blood–brain barrier, and thus affect water permeability, might therefore be expected to alter the shape of the residue function. However, for practical purposes, the effects of restrictions on water exchange are expected to be small, primarily owing to the high inherent permeability of water that is expected, but also owing to the small difference in T_1 between capillary blood (shorter than arterial blood, but longer than tissue) and the extravascular "tissue." The possibility of using ASL to measure permeability is discussed in Box 4.10.

Box 4.10: **Measuring permeability using ASL**

Efforts to probe and exploit changes in water permeability and exchange in ASL tend to center on methods that can amplify differences between label in blood and label in tissue. These proceed generally either by using flow crushers to distinguish between labeled water that is stationary in the tissue (i.e., has been delivered) and (slowly) moving capillary blood water, or by varying the echo time to derive a T_2 weighting to detect water that is in different environments (vascular versus extravascular) based on differing T_2 between the environments. These methods are very much research tools and not widely used currently.

4.6 Accelerated decay: modeling a low-flip-angle readout

As noted in Section 2.3, one approach to acquiring ASL data at multiple PLDs is to use a Look-Locker readout. The use of small flip angles retains some of the signal at one PLD, which can be measured later at the next PLD. The effect of doing this is to reduce the signal magnitude at each readout by a small amount. For the purposes of kinetic analysis, this looks as if the decay of the labeled water is happening more rapidly than the T_1 value would suggest. We can model this by using a corrected T_1 value; see Box 4.11.

> ### Box 4.11: A modified T_1 decay relationship for Look–Locker readouts
>
> The effect of Look–Locker pulses on the magnitude of the ASL label–control difference signal can be approximated by assuming that T_1 decay has been accelerated according to the formula
>
> $$1/T_1' = 1/T_1 - \log(\cos(FA))/\delta PLD$$
>
> where
>
> T_1' is the corrected T_1 decay rate that can be used to describe the T_1 in the kinetic model,
> FA is the flip angle of the Look–Locker pulses, and
> δPLD is the time between acquisition of each PLD.

4.7 Quantifying perfusion

The purpose of developing a kinetic model for ASL data was so that we could relate measured signal to perfusion, to enable us to make quantitative measurements. Thus far, we have developed a model that, for a given perfusion value, predicts the ASL difference signal. The final thing we need to do is convert this model so that, for a given measured difference signal in a voxel, we get a perfusion value. For single-PLD data, the conversion step can simply be performed by rearranging the equation of the kinetic model and producing a formula that can then be applied. For multi-PLD data, a little more work is required, and we need methods that produce a best fit of the model to the data. One option that we will consider further in this chapter is Bayesian inference. This approach works very neatly for both single- and multi-PLD data and brings with it a number of other advantages when applied to perfusion estimation using ASL.

4.7.1 Perfusion quantification formulae

The simplest model we met in Section 4.1 converts to the formula provided by the consensus paper for quantification of pcASL with a single PLD; see Box 1.3. A similar equation can be derived for pASL, where it is assumed that the label duration is known (set by QUIPSS II pulses); see Box 4.12. Critically, to apply these equations, we need to be sampling in the tail of the kinetic curve, where we are minimally sensitive to ATT; thus, there is a limit on the ATT, beyond which the equation becomes inaccurate; see Box 4.4.

Box 4.12: Quantifying perfusion from pASL data using the simple model

The consensus paper gives the formula for quantifying perfusion from pASL data (with QUIPSS II to define the label duration) as

$$CBF = \frac{6000\lambda(S_{control} - S_{label})e^{TI/T_1}}{2\alpha \cdot TI_1 \cdot S_{PD}}$$

where

$S_{control} - S_{label}$ is the result of label–control subtraction,
S_{PD} is the magnitude of the proton-density-weighted image,
TI is the inversion time,
TI_1 is the timing of the QUIPSS II pulse and sets the label duration (the recommended value is 800 ms).

A standard value of T_1 for arterial blood is recommended, taken from the literature to be 1.65 s at 3 T, together with a standard value of the pASL labeling efficiency α of 0.98 and a single whole-brain partition coefficient value λ of 0.9.

The standard model can be converted in a similar way to the simple model. The standard model is a strictly non-linear function of perfusion owing to the appearance of perfusion in the residue function through the outflow effect. However, the effect of perfusion on the residue function is quite small, so, to a first approximation, we can assume in that term that it takes a fixed value, say 0.01 s^{-1} (60 ml/100g/min) without introducing substantial bias. Owing to the presence of the outflow term, it is also necessary to specify a value for the partition coefficient, for which the value for brain (mixed gray and white matter) of 0.9 is often used.

4.7.2 Model fitting

When dealing with multi-PLD data, model fitting is required because we have measurements at different points in the kinetic curve and we need to account for the different information each measurement gives about perfusion via the model. Typically, the purpose of multi-PLD data is to account for the variability of other parameters in the kinetic model, such as ATT, the aim being the estimation of perfusion and other parameters from the model. In practice, you will find either that software for analyzing ASL data simply does not offer the option to handle multi-PLD ASL or that it has made a specific choice as to what model fitting method to use, although you may be able to adjust some fitting parameters if you are having problems with your data.

Since the model is nonlinear in at least some of the parameters, ATT being a notable one, a nonlinear algorithm is required. Most widely used nonlinear least-squares methods are based on a variant of the Gauss–Newton approach. As in linear regression, the idea is to minimize the squared error between the model-fit and the data. This makes the assumption that the noise on the data is white, which is a reasonable approximation for most ASL data. Because the model is nonlinear, the Gauss–Newton approach performs the minimization iteratively and bases the next guess of the parameters on a linear approximation to the function at the current estimate (using a Taylor expansion). The combination of linear approximations and nonlinear model can make the convergence of the fit to the optimal solution tricky, and most implementations include various modifications that aim to improve this and may also offer the ability to apply limits on the parameter values. An alternative to model fitting that is sometimes applicable to ASL data is "model-free" deconvolution as discussed in Box 4.13.

Box 4.13: Model-free deconvolution

A noted in Section 4.1, the fundamental model for ASL data involves the convolution of two functions: the arterial input and residue functions. Typically for ASL analysis, we assume parameterized functional forms for each and seek to set the parameters from the acquisition or estimate them from the data or using literature sources. This means that the result can be somewhat dependent upon information that does not hold in the given individual being scanned. For example, T_1 might vary substantially in pathological tissue, or the specified bolus duration could not be achieved. The ideal, therefore, would be to get more individual specific information from the data. One approach to do this is to try to estimate the AIF directly. This is already quite common in other perfusion imaging methods, but requires extra effort in ASL. It is necessary to capture specifically signal in major arteries, which is often achieved using flow suppression to isolate the "tissue" signal and through subtraction calculate a voxelwise arterial signal; this is the rationale behind the QUASAR sequence (see Box 2.12).

If you have an estimated AIF, it is then possible to use it to directly estimate the residue function from the tissue signal, and with it the perfusion. This process is often referred to as deconvolution, the reversal of the convolution present in the model. Unfortunately, this process is also poorly conditioned, although various solutions exist to make it possible to obtain estimates of the residue function even when faced with the noise common in ASL data. This is still a very specialized solution for ASL analysis, since it requires specific choices to be made when the data is acquired. However, its greatest strength is the potential to deal with the effects of dispersion (see Section 4.4), since the measured AIFs are normally local to the tissue where deconvolution is performed and thus have already experienced the effects of dispersion.

4.7.3 Bayesian inversion

An alternative approach is to cast the model inversion problem as one of Bayesian inference. The essence of this, when applied to ASL, is that instead of seeking a single value as an estimate for each parameter in the model, we seek a probability distribution that captures the uncertainty in our estimate of the parameter given the data we have. From this distribution, we can extract classical statistical measures such as the mean (a best "guess" at the parameter value) and variance (a measure of uncertainty around the mean). By recasting parameters as distributions, we also have the ability to include information in our data analysis about the parameters from before we collected the data—via the "prior" distributions. What this allows us to do is utilize any knowledge that we have about the parameter values that is separate from the ASL data itself. For example, ATT is something we might want to estimate from the data, since it will vary within the brain. However, it is a parameter that is fairly well limited by physiology, so we can use our prior distribution to capture the plausible range of values that ATT might take. Another example is T_1, something that we typically set based on a literature value, but which is known to vary from individual to individual and within an individual. We can incorporate into the prior on T_1 not only the "normal" literature value, but also a degree of variability. The range of prior information in ASL is illustrated in Figure 4.10.

The prior information that we have discussed so far is "biophysical" in origin, but there is a further source of information that we might want to exploit, namely, spatial homogeneity. We are interested in using ASL to map perfusion, and we know that ASL is noisy, but also that perfusion varies relatively smoothly from one region of the brain to another—certainly over the scale of voxels within an ASL image. Thus, we should be able to exploit this inherent smoothness, or similarity between neighboring voxels, to improve our results. One approach is to smooth the data as discussed in Chapter 3. However, that involves making an arbitrary decision about the amount of smoothing we want. It is also problematic for multi-PLD ASL if we combine data from voxels with different ATTs, since it is possible that the resulting time course will no longer

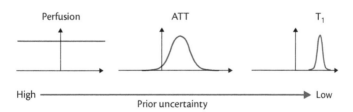

Figure 4.10: An illustration of the prior information applied to typical ASL parameters. Here we are showing that there are some parameters, such as T_1, that we wish to constrain based on information we have about the parameter, whereas for perfusion we would like information from this to arise only from the ASL data we have collected. We might want to exclude negative values for all these parameters and adjust the distributions accordingly. Whether we can do this in practice depends upon the algorithm we are using.

resemble the expected kinetic curve shape, hindering accurate fitting. Bayesian inference offers an alternative solution, whereby we encode the spatial relationships within a spatial prior. The perfusion estimate in any voxel is now informed by the values of its neighbors, but, being "prior" information, this will play more or less of a role in the estimation depending upon how informative the data in that voxel is. Thus, in regions of high noise, smoother perfusion estimates will be obtained, but in lower-noise regions, spatial features in the perfusion image will still appear. Thus, the use of a spatial prior is inherently "adaptive," adjusting the effective degree of smoothing based on the data itself.

SUMMARY

- A kinetic model is required to relate measured image intensity to delivery of labeled blood-water and thereby perfusion.

- Kinetic models for ASL describe both the delivery of the labeled blood-water and also the decay of the label, using the convolution of the arterial input and residue functions.

- The simplest model for ASL kinetics neglects ATT, assuming that the measurements that are made are insensitive to this parameter.

- An arterial component can be included in the model to account for labeled blood-water still in the larger vessels at the time of imaging.

- Dispersion of the labeled blood-water bolus during transit through the vasculature can be included in the model and will affect the overall quantification of perfusion.

- Multi-PLD data allows more parameters of the model to be estimated and thus a more accurate measure of perfusion as well as information about hemodynamics to be obtained. This process requires some form of model fitting or Bayesian inference method.

FURTHER READING

- Buxton, R. B., Frank, L. R., Wong, E. C., Siewert, B., Warach, S., & Edelman, R. R. (1998). A general kinetic model for quantitative perfusion imaging with arterial spin labeling. *Magnetic Resonance in Medicine, 40*, 383–396.
    - *This is the classic paper that describes the general tracer kinetic model as applied to ASL. It introduces what we have called here the "standard" model and also discusses the limitations and potential extensions of this model.*
- Hrabe, J. & Lewis, D. (2004). Two analytical solutions for a model of pulsed arterial spin labeling with randomized blood arrival times. *Journal of Magnetic Resonance, 167*, 49–55.

- *This is a good example of a vascular transport function-based modification of the standard model to account for dispersion. It also includes a good formulation of the standard model and how it may be derived from the Bloch equations.*

- Chappell, M. A., MacIntosh, B. J., Donahue, M. J., Günther, M., Jezzard, P. & Woolrich, M. W. (2010). Separation of macrovascular signal in multi-inversion time arterial spin labeling MRI. *Magnetic Resonance in Medicine*, 63, 1357–1365.
  - *An example of the use of an additional macrovascular component in the model to account for labeled blood-water still in major arteries and a comparison of this approach with flow suppression.*

- Chappell, M. A. Woolrich, M. W. Kazan, S., Jezzard, P., Payne, S. J. & MacIntosh, B. J. (2013). Modeling dispersion in arterial spin labeling: validation using dynamic angiographic measurements. *Magnetic Resonance in Medicine*, 69, 563–570.
  - *This work compares a range of different models for dispersion of ASL labeled blood-water, looking specifically at data from arterial blood using an angiographic readout.*

- Petersen, E., Lim, T. & Golay, X. (2006). Model-free arterial spin labeling quantification approach for perfusion MRI. *Magnetic Resonance in Medicine*, 55, 219–232.
  - *In this work, the "model-free," deconvolution approach to solving the tracer kinetic model for perfusion imaging is applied for the first time to ASL data, using a specific (QUASAR) sequence designed to provide independent measures of arterial and tissue ASL signal.*

- Chappell, M. A., Woolrich, M. W., Petersen, E. T., Golay, X. & Payne, S. J. (2013). Comparing model based and model-free analysis methods for QUASAR arterial spin labeling perfusion quantification. *Magnetic Resonance in Medicine*, 69, 1466–1475.
  - *This provides a comparison of "model-free" deconvolution and model fitting analysis for QUASAR ASL, including the effects of dispersion.*

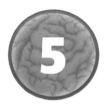

Calibration: Estimating Arterial Blood Magnetization

The key to absolute quantification of perfusion using ASL is knowledge of the concentration of the labeled blood-water tracer, and this is achieved by estimation of the magnetization of arterial blood. It is this quantity that appears as the amplitude of the arterial input function of the kinetic model (see, e.g., Boxes 4.2 and 4.3). Without this, the images remain in the arbitrary units of the signal from the scanner, but with an estimate of this parameter, it is possible to quote perfusion in absolute units of ml/100 g/min.

More precisely, we need the magnetization of arterial blood where (and when) the labeling was performed. There are broadly two schools of thought as to how this value should be determined: either it is estimated *voxelwise*, in every single voxel of the image, from the magnetization of the tissue, or a single global value is estimated by taking the mean over a *reference region*. The argument for the reference region approach is that since we expect a single value of magnetization for the arterial blood as it is passing through the labeling plane, we cannot have a different value in every voxel. The argument for a voxelwise approach is that this might be able to automatically correct for other voxelwise variations in intensity such as coil sensitivity (see Section 2.4), and it is also typically an easier calculation to make. For these reasons the consensus paper has recommended the voxelwise method for general purpose calibration.

5.1 The partition coefficient

Both methods assume that the magnetization of arterial blood can be related to that in brain tissue (or cerebrospinal fluid, CSF) via the partition coefficient:

$$M_{0b} = M_{0t} / \lambda$$

where λ is taken to be the classical partition coefficient from the positron emission tomography (PET) literature relating the density of water in tissue to that in blood (see Box 5.1). The units of

λ are quoted as either ml blood/ml tissue or ml blood/g tissue, the latter being more useful for perfusion quantification if we are aiming for units of ml blood/100g tissue/min. Typical values used in ASL perfusion quantification are given in Table 5.1.

Box 5.1: What is the partition coefficient?

The units of λ can be confusing, since it is strictly a dimensionless quantity, being a ratio of densities:

$$\lambda = \rho_t / \rho_b$$

where

ρ_t is the density of water in tissue and
ρ_b is the density of water in blood.

Thus, it is common to explicitly quote the two species involved, in this case tissue and blood. This can cause further confusion, since the units appear to be the "wrong way up": the ratio has tissue on the top of the fraction, but the units have blood on top. This is resolved by considering the full units of the equation:

$$\lambda = \frac{g\,H_2O/ml\,tissue}{g\,H_2O\,/ml\,blood} = \frac{ml\,blood}{ml\,tissue}$$

The use of a value for λ derived from the PET literature might not be strictly accurate for ASL quantification, since we might not see some pools of water that are visible in a radiotracer experiment, for example, pools of bound water with short T_2 that are responsible for magnetization transfer effects. The correct value of λ would thus be smaller than that commonly quoted. This is an argument in favor of a reference region approach using CSF for calibration, since CSF is a watery fluid and there are less likely to be pools that are invisible to MR acquisition. For this reason, as well as to minimize issues of partial voluming, the CSF only in the ventricles is normally used for calibration purposes.

5.2 Equilibrium magnetization

For calibration, it is thus necessary to estimate the magnetization of some or all brain tissue. The ideal data for this is an image with a long TR (compared with the T_1 of the tissues), which is commonly called a proton-density-weighted image since it is predominantly a measure of water content and not other physical properties (such as T_1). If background suppression has been applied, there will be reduced static tissue signal remaining in the ASL data, and a separate acquisition, without background suppression, is often needed for calibration purposes. Corrections for shorter TR or other manipulations, such as pre-saturation of the imaging region, are also possible. For example, the consensus paper recommends the following correction for TR less than 5 s:

$$1/(1 - e^{-TR/T_1})$$

Table 5.1 Typical values of the partition coefficient for brain tissues as used in ASL perfusion quantification.

Tissue	Value ml blood/ml tissue
Whole brain*	0.9
Gray matter	0.98
White matter	0.82
CSF	1.15

* Effectively the mean of gray and white matter and used where a mixture of the tissues is expected.

Source: data from Herscovitch, P. & Raichle, M. E., 'What is the correct value for the brain–blood partition coefficient for water?', *Journal of Cerebral Blood Flow and Metabolism*, Volume 5, Issue 1, pp. 65–69, DOI: 10.1038/jcbfm.1985.9, Copyright © 1985 SAGE Publications.

where T_1 is that of the tissue. In the absence of background suppression, an approximate calibration image can be obtained from the static tissue images; for example, the control images can sometimes be used for this, since the contribution of the perfusion signal is small. Complications can arise where other aspects of the ASL preparation or readout also affect the control image magnitude; see Box 5.2. An illustration of calibration using the voxelwise approach is given in Example Box 5.1.

Box 5.2: The magnetization of tissue under different preparations or readouts

There are a range of different preparations that may be combined with ASL, largely with the view of reducing the static tissue signal. The major ones are considered here to show that it is still possible to extract magnetization estimates from the static tissue signal; in some cases, it is even possible to get extra images such as a T_1 map that can be included in the main analysis. Some of these preparations might be used to achieve background suppression, but other more advanced schemes are often used that do not lend themselves to estimation of arterial blood magnetization.

Without pre-saturation

In a conventional readout, the static tissue signal in any voxel (once a steady state has been achieved) can be related to the magnetization by

$$S = M_0(1 - e^{-TR/T_1})$$

where T_1 is that of the static tissue (and T_2 decay is being ignored).

This accounts for partial saturation due to the TR and can simply be solved to estimate a voxelwise M_0 value for the static tissue. This is the basis of the consensus paper recommendation for short-TR images.

With pre-saturation

If pre-saturation of the imaging region is performed, typically just before the start of labeling, then the relationship between signal and equilibrium magnetization becomes

$$S = M_0(1 - Ae^{-t/T_{1t}})$$

where

    t is the time from saturation to imaging and
    A is the saturation efficiency.

A multi-PLD acquisition will provide a range of samples from the saturation recovery curve, from which M_0, A and T_{1t} can be determined by model fitting, in a similar way to a sampled kinetic curve.

Look–Locker readout with pre-saturation

For the case of a Look–Locker type of multi-PLD acquisition, it is also necessary to account for the effects of the low-flip-angle readout pulses. In this case, the signal equation becomes

$$S = M'_{0t}(1 - Ae^{-t/T'_{1t}})$$

where

    $M'_{0t} = M_{0t}(1 - e^{-\delta TI/T_{1t}})/(1 - \cos(FA)e^{-\delta TI/T_{1t}})$,

    $1/T'_{1t} = 1/T_{1t} - \log(\cos(FA))/\delta TI$,

FA is the flip angle, and
δTI is the interval between inversion times.
Here the approximation from Box 4.11 has been used.

Example Box 5.1: Voxelwise calibration

For the single-PLD data in Chapter 1 we applied voxelwise calibration and obtained the absolute perfusion image in Figure 1.7; this was using the calibration image shown on the left of Figure 5.1. We can now update that result using the spatial prior regularization we met in Chapter 4 to give the perfusion image on the left of Figure 5.2, which still has the issue we noted in Example Box 1.3 of artifactual values around the edge of the brain due to the low intensity of the calibration image in voxels that are only partially filled with brain tissue. For the perfusion image shown on the right of Figure 5.2, we have addressed this issue using a simple procedure:

- Median filtering—a spatial filtering operation that smoothes out noise in the image.
- Erosion of voxels around the edge of the brain (based on the mask created when processing the data), shown in the center of Figure 5.1.

■ Extrapolation to refill the voxels we have eroded using the remaining values within the brain, shown on the right of Figure 5.1. To perform the extrapolation, we have taken the average of non-zero values within an ROI centered on the empty voxel that we want to fill.

This procedure works on the basis that we expect the calibration image, which is approximately a proton-density-weighted image, to be smoothly varying, and thus the errors introduced by extrapolation are likely to be far smaller than those due to partial voluming.

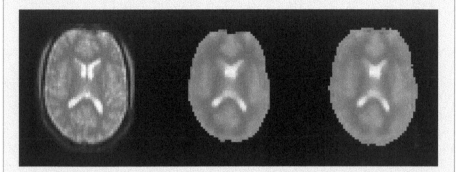

Figure 5.1: Calibration image for the single-PLD data introduced in Chapter 1 (left). This has been smoothed with a median spatial filter and eroded to remove voxels around the edge of the brain that are only partially filled with brain tissue (center) and then extrapolated to refill the removed voxels with values based on those remaining (right), to produce a corrected calibration image.

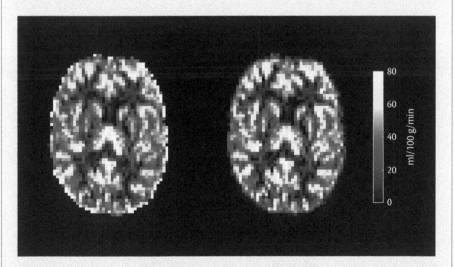

Figure 5.2: Absolute perfusion image for the single PLD data of Chapter 1 using voxelwise calibration (left) and after correction for partial volume effects around the edge of the brain (right).

5.3 Generating a reference region

The most common reference regions are ventricular CSF or white matter. In both cases, it is most accurate to use as the reference region a region of interest (ROI) that contains only voxels of pure CSF or white matter (and thus gray matter is a bad choice for the reference region because of the low resolution of the ASL acquisition; see Chapter 6). Apart from manual delineation of the ROI, the reference region can be obtained using automated segmentation:

- Segmentation of a high-resolution structural image with subsequent transformation of the partial volume estimates into the low resolution of the ASL data before thresholding at a high value to create a mask with minimal contamination at the boundaries.

- Segmentation of a low-resolution T_1 image derived from saturation recovery fitting to the ASL data, where pre-saturation has been used with a multi-PLD acquisition.

The former method is more universal, since it can be performed with any ASL acquisition. A high-resolution structural image must be acquired separately, but this is quite common and recommended in general for registration purposes, especially in group studies. However, it does rely on a good registration between ASL data and the structural image, something that we considered in Chapter 3. The generation of a CSF-based reference region is illustrated in Example Box 5.2.

Example Box 5.2: A CSF-based reference region

The calibration carried out to produce the "best" analysis in Chapter 1 (see Example Box 1.3), plus those for the pcASL data in Chapter 4, were carried out using the ventricular CSF in the calibration image as a reference. The automatically generated ventricle mask is shown in Figure 5.3, and this was derived from a segmentation of the structural image, followed by masking with the locations of the ventricles from the Harvard–Oxford Atlas, before transformation into the resolution of the ASL data.

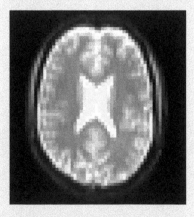

Figure 5.3: Automatically generated ventricular mask within which the magnetization of CSF was calculated from the calibration image.

5.4 T_2 or T_2^* correction

Since the data will have been acquired at a non-zero echo time, a correction can be made for T_2 or T_2^* decay. Whether this needs to be a correction for T_2 or T_2^* will depend upon the acquisition; see Chapter 2. For the voxelwise approach, the equilibrium magnetization of arterial blood is effectively being estimated in the same voxel as the perfusion, so the effects of T_2 or T_2^* decay on the static tissue will be similar to that on the blood, and therefore this effect is often disregarded. For the reference region approach, the T_2 or T_2^* of the reference region might vary substantially from that in any given voxel, and therefore correction may be warranted using the formulae in Box 5.3.

Box 5.3: Correcting for differences in T_2 or T_2^*

The equilibrium magnetization of arterial blood, M'_{0a} will be related to the M_0 estimated from the static tissue/reference region by

$$M_{0a} = \frac{M_0}{\lambda} e^{TE/T_2}$$

where T_2 here is that of the tissue/reference region. Correction for the T_2 decay of the perfusion data itself can be achieved by incorporating this into the value for the equilibrium magnetization of arterial blood that we will use for the final quantification:

$$M'_{0a} = M_{0a} e^{-TE/T_2}$$

where T_2 here is that for the what the labeled blood-water experienced during the acquisition—somewhere between the arterial or capillary blood and tissue values. The same procedure follows for T_2^*, with the relevant T_2 values being replaced by those of T_2^*.

5.5 Quantifying perfusion

As we saw in Section 2.6, it might be necessary to correct for the effects of coil sensitivity on the ASL data. In principle, the voxelwise method for calculation of arterial blood magnetization inherently contains a correction for this effect, since both the ASL images and the calibration image are affected in the same way. For the reference region approach, this is not the case and—particularly for a CSF reference region at the center of the image—sensitivity correction may have a noticeable effect on the quantified perfusion values. In this case, a correction for coil sensitivity needs to be applied to both the ASL data and the calibration image before arterial blood magnetization is estimated and perfusion quantified. You might also need to be alert to deliberately applied global scaling differences between the ASL data and the calibration image; see Box 5.4.

Box 5.4: Acquisition gain settings

One thing that hopefully will have become clear is that there is normally a difference of approximately two orders of magnitude in signal between the calibration image and the label–control difference images. To increase the accuracy with which this smaller signal is measured, sometimes the person who setup the ASL sequence will choose a different gain setting, or magnitude scaling, for the calibration image compared with the main ASL data, particularly when background suppression is being used. Doing this is helpful, since it can reduce errors associated with the conversion from an analog signal to the digital value stored in the computer. However, if this has happened, you need to be aware of it and scale the resulting images to make them match; otherwise the quantified perfusion values will be wrong.

An estimate of arterial blood magnetization gives a measure of the "concentration" of the label created in the labeling region. However, in practice, this labeling will not be 100% efficient and thus the magnetization of the labeled blood will be lower than the ideal case, as we saw in Section 2.1. Thus, the value needs to be corrected by the inversion efficiency. It may be possible to measure this on an individual basis (although that measurement will have its own sources of error), and this might be considered when using pcASL in a population where variations in arterial flow velocity are expected. However, it is far more typical to use standard values for inversion efficiency, and the consensus paper recommends values of 0.98 for pASL and 0.85 for pcASL.

Finally, the corrected estimate for the arterial blood magnetization can be used with the result of kinetic modeling to provide quantitative perfusion measurements. For the simplest cases, the process of estimating and applying the arterial blood magnetization is built into the formula used for quantification, along with the kinetic model. This is what we have seen in the consensus paper formulae in Box 1.3 for pcASL and Box 4.12 for pASL. Some analysis software might separate the two processes, doing the kinetic modeling first to produce a relative perfusion value, corrected for the tracer kinetics, and then perform a division of this value by the estimated blood magnetization (either as an image or a single value) as a further step. This allows you flexibility to use a different calibration method, should you find that one has failed for some reason, without having to repeat the whole analysis.

An illustration of the use of a reference region versus voxelwise calibration is given in Example Box 5.3.

Example Box 5.3: Reference region versus voxelwise calibration

Figure 5.4 compares the final perfusion image for the data from Chapter 1 when using the CSF as a reference to calculate the magnetization of arterial blood or using the calibration image directly to perform voxelwise calibration. Reassuringly, the two images are very similar and the choice of calibration process has not made much difference in this case.

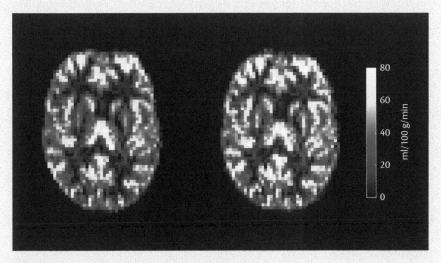

Figure 5.4: Quantified perfusion (in ml/100 g/min) in the middle slice of the pcASL data from Chapter 1 using CSF as a reference region (left) or voxelwise calibration (right).

On the primer website, you will find the data used in the examples in this chapter, along with instructions on how to perform both voxelwise-based and CSF reference-region-based calibration.

SUMMARY

- Calibration, the process of obtaining a perfusion value in absolute units of ml/100 g/min, involves the calculation of the value of the equilibrium magnetization of arterial blood.
- Calibration can be performed on a voxelwise basis or by obtaining a single value from a reference region.
- For the reference region approach, ventricular CSF or white matter both represent choices that allow for robust estimates with minimal partial volume effects.

FURTHER READING

- *Precise details of the calibration process used with ASL data can often be tricky to find in the literature, since this information is often buried in the methods or omitted altogether. The following are papers that include specific recommendations or relevant theory.*

- Alsop, D. C., Detre, J. A., Golay, X., Günther, M., Hendrikse, J., Hernandez-Garcia, L., et al. (2015). Recommended implementation of arterial spin-labeled perfusion MRI for clinical applications: A consensus of the ISMRM Perfusion Study Group and the European Consortium for ASL in Dementia. *Magnetic Resonance in Medicine*, 73, 102–116.
  - *The consensus paper advocates the use of voxelwise calibration as a simple and universal way of arriving at fully quantified perfusion images from ASL.*

- Chappell, M. A., Woolrich, M. W., Petersen, E. T., Golay, X. & Payne, S. J. (2013). Comparing model-based and model-free analysis methods for QUASAR arterial spin labeling perfusion quantification. *Magnetic Resonance in Medicine*, 69, 1466–1475.
  - *This work includes details relating to the use of saturation recovery data for calibration of ASL data; it specifically considers the QUASAR sequence, but the principles can be applied more broadly.*

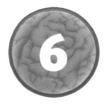

Partial Volume Effects

Partial volume (PV) effects can be very substantial in the quantification of perfusion using ASL. The problem arises partially from the low resolution of ASL data compared to the dimensions of the white/gray matter structure of the brain. Since gray matter predominantly forms a relatively thin, highly folded sheet, and the dimensions of a typical ASL voxel are of the order of 3 mm, most cortical voxels contain some mixture of gray matter, white matter, and/or CSF. Figure 6.1 shows gray and white matter partial volume estimates from a high-resolution structural image that has been segmented. These partial volumes have then been projected onto an image with a typical ASL resolution of 3 mm × 3 mm × 5 mm, then thresholded at 90% to reveal regions of "pure" gray and white matter. Notice, particularly for gray matter, how few voxels can be considered pure at the resolution of ASL data.

The other reason why partial volume effects are an issue for ASL is the different perfusion properties of the different brain tissues. Gray matter is regarded as having a typical perfusion of 60 ml/100g/min, whereas white matter is expected to be nearer to 20 ml/100g/min and CSF has zero perfusion. Thus, the apparent perfusion in any given voxel is likely to depend strongly upon the contents of that voxel. This effect can be seen when you compare a perfusion image alongside the matching image of gray matter partial volume, as shown in Figure 6.2. There is a remarkable similarity between the visual appearance of both, reflecting the fact that it is the gray matter that dominates the perfusion image. This means that the measured perfusion in any voxel is a combination of the perfusion of gray matter (and, to a lesser extent, white matter) at that location multiplied by the proportion of the voxel taken up by gray matter. In effect, a perfusion image contains perfusion information modulated on top of a structural image.

6.1 PV effects and mean gray matter perfusion

It is common to use ASL data to calculate the mean gray matter perfusion, and very often you will see this value reported in the literature. This will be done by generating a gray matter mask

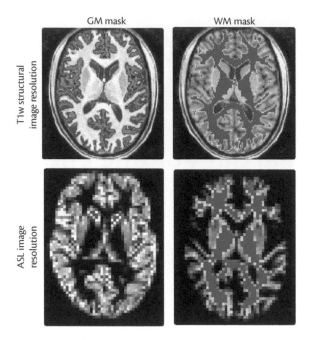

Figure 6.1: Illustration of the effects of partial voluming on the occurrence of voxels with a high proportion of gray or white matter at the resolution of a typical structural image (1 mm in-plane) and an ASL image (3 mm in-plane). Here gray and white matter masks have been created at both resolutions using a threshold of 90% PV.

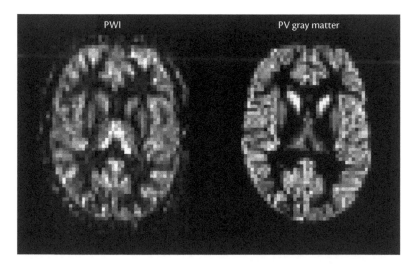

Figure 6.2: A comparison of an ASL perfusion-weighted image (PWI) alongside the anatomical PV estimates of gray matter (at the same resolution) shows that both visually share a lot of similar "structure."

and averaging within the mask. However, the manner in which this mask is created can substantially affect the mean gray matter value calculated, largely as a result of PV effects. Figure 6.1 gives an extreme example of a gray matter mask where we have attempted to use a very high threshold to get pure gray matter, but we are left with very few voxels, and so our mean gray matter perfusion value will not be robust to noise. If we lowered the threshold, we would include more voxels in the mask, but would therefore also be including a greater proportion of non-gray-matter tissue. Figure 6.3 shows, in a typical ASL perfusion image, how the mean gray and white matter perfusion vary with the threshold used to create the mask. Notice that as the threshold gets higher, we tend toward the "expected" values for each tissue type, and in general we tend to underestimate gray matter perfusion (and overestimate white matter perfusion). This explains (at least partially) why whole-brain gray matter perfusion estimates from ASL are often lower than the expected 60 ml blood/100g tissue/min, since, even if we attempt to segment the gray matter to make an ROI over which to take the mean, we are going to include many voxels that are partially white matter and CSF. If we try to be very strict about our definition of a gray matter voxel, we run into the problems of Figure 6.1 and have too few voxels to get a meaningful perfusion estimate. We can also get a different answer if we apply the threshold to the PV estimate in the original space of the structural image or to the ASL data; see Box 6.1.

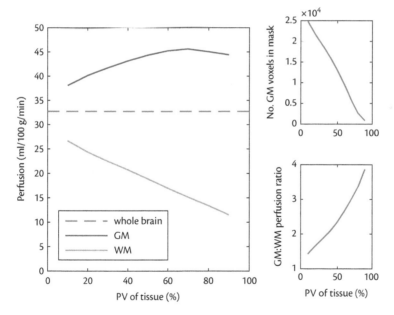

Figure 6.3: Mean perfusion calculated in gray and white matter from an ASL dataset in which the threshold used to generate the gray matter or white matter mask has been varied. A higher threshold leads to larger mean gray matter perfusion and lower mean white matter perfusion values. Also shown is the variation in the number of voxels included in the gray matter mask as the gray matter PV threshold is raised, along with the variation in the ratio of gray to white matter.

Box 6.1: **Thresholding PV estimate maps to make masks**

For Figure 6.1, we deliberately transformed the PV effect from the high-resolution image to the low resolution of the ASL data *before* applying a threshold. It is tempting to threshold at the high resolution to create a mask (or accept the gray matter mask produced by the segmentation method, based on the tissue type with the highest PV in the voxel) and then transform that to the ASL data space. However, these two processes typically arrive at different solutions owing to interpolation, as shown in Figure 6.4. Note that once you transform a mask, you have to apply another (arbitrary) threshold to get back to a binary mask; in this case, we used 0.7 again.

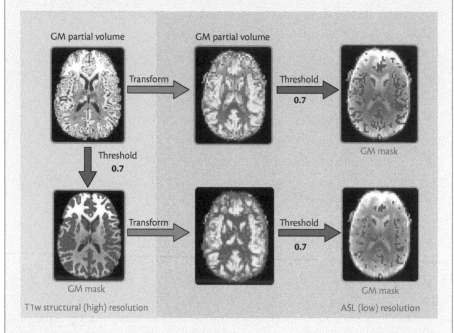

Figure 6.4: The choice of when to threshold the gray matter PV image when creating a gray matter mask can make a noticeable difference to the mask generated and hence to any values computed using that mask.

The effects we have observed reflect what will be happening in the voxel, with a partial combination of gray and white matter leading to an overestimate of perfusion for white matter in the voxel but an underestimate for gray matter, with any CSF reducing the perfusion overall. If we simply treat the ASL signal as being an estimator of gray matter perfusion (since white matter is somewhat smaller), we will routinely arrive at an underestimate. An illustration of calculating mean perfusion values in brain tissue is given in Example Box 6.1.

Example Box 6.1: Mean perfusion in gray and white matter

Using a T_1-weighted anatomical image acquired at the same time as the ASL data in Chapter 1, we can compute gray and white matter ROIs and thereby compute the mean perfusion with each tissue type to be as follows:

gray matter: 41.0 ml/100 g/min
white matter: 10.3 ml/100 g/min

For these calculations, the ROIs were defined from PV estimates that had been transformed to the same resolution as the ASL data using a threshold of 70% for the gray matter and 90% for the white matter. The ROIs (including tissue masks generated using a threshold of 10% PV of tissue) are shown in Figure 6.5 alongside the perfusion image.

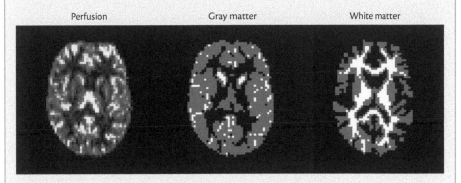

Figure 6.5: The perfusion image from the single-PLD data from Chapter 1 with "pure" tissue ROI (in white) for gray matter (center) and white matter (right) using a threshold of 90% of that tissue type; these are overlaid on a tissue mask ROI thresholded at 10% (in gray color) for reference.

6.2 PV correction

If we assume that we can make reasonable estimates of the partial volumes of white matter, gray matter, and CSF within each ASL voxel (see the primer in this series "Introduction to Neuroimaging Analysis" for more on segmentation methodology, and also Box 6.2 for a discussion on what we mean by white and gray matter in this context), the question is whether we can calculate pure gray matter (and possibly white matter) perfusion from our ASL data. The problem is that in each voxel we only have measures of combined perfusion, but we want to separate out two sources of perfusion. In our typical single-PLD ASL experiment, we only have a single measurement of the difference signal. While we might have made this measurement repeatedly to improve SNR, these extra measurements give us no new information about the separation of gray and white matter perfusion. We need to get some more information from somewhere. One option is to exploit the extra information provided by multi-PLD ASL data, a topic which we will return to. A simpler approach is to assume either a fixed value for white matter perfusion or a fixed ratio between gray and white matter perfusion (3:1 being an expected ratio). Both of these make a strict assumption that is unlikely to be true everywhere in the brain, and certainly not in pathology. Thus, although it is simple to implement and has been used in studies, this approach is not recommended.

Box 6.2: What do we mean by gray and white matter?

The issue of PV effects is common across all neuroimaging methods, but is particularly problematic in perfusion imaging because white matter has been observed to have much lower perfusion than gray matter, reflecting the different role it plays in the brain. However, how reasonable is it, for the purposes of perfusion and other hemodynamics, to divide the brain neatly into white and gray matter?

Our working definition of the two tissue types in neuroimaging is effectively driven by the differences observed on structural imaging. These are supported by histological studies of the brain that show that what we call gray and white matter are distinctly different; see the primer in this series "Introduction to Neuroimaging Analysis." In reality, though, there is more variability than just the two tissue types: for example in the layered structure of the cortex, there are details that we cannot typically observe with non-invasive neuroimaging methods. Thus, the gray matter observed in one voxel could be very different from the gray matter observed in another voxel. To a great extent, this is not problematic for perfusion imaging, since it deliberately seeks to measure perfusion within individual voxels without making assumptions about the tissue. It may be more problematic for PV correction, since we use imaging-derived measures of gray and white matter proportion to define "pure" gray (and white) matter perfusion measurements.

The implications of this are mainly interpretative: we have to accept that (at the moment anyway) when we use PV correction to extract gray matter perfusion, the value we will obtain in any given voxel corresponds to whatever tissue has been classed as gray matter by our PV estimation method. This might not be the same physical combination of cells as elsewhere in the brain, but hopefully will be consistent between individuals. Importantly, this highlights that, at the very least, PV-corrected perfusion is reliant on the consistency of the PV estimates.

6.2.1 Using spatial information

The other option for obtaining more information is to stop treating voxels in isolation and instead incorporate information about the local neighborhood into our estimation procedure. We will make the assumption that the perfusion varies slowly in space compared with the resolution of our voxels, i.e., that the perfusion image should vary minimally as we move from one voxel to another. This seems physiologically plausible, although there might be regions and cases where we might want to preserve more sharply defined features in the perfusion image.

The simplest way to incorporate this information is via a method based on linear regression; see Box 6.3 for more details. This method defines a kernel in which we assume that both white matter and gray matter perfusion is identical in all voxels. We center this kernel on a voxel and, using all the voxels in the kernel, estimate gray and white matter difference signals and assign the values to that voxel. We proceed through all the voxels in the brain. Often a 2D kernel in-plane (i.e., the axial plane) is specified, reflecting the non-isotropic voxel dimensions of most ASL data, although 3D kernels are also valid.

Box 6.3: Linear regression for PV correction

We can write the ASL label–control difference signal as

$$\Delta M = PV_{GM} \cdot \Delta M_{GM} + PV_{WM} \cdot \Delta M_{WM} + PV_{CSF} \cdot \Delta M_{CSF}$$

where

ΔM_x is the label–control difference signal from tissue x and
PV_x is the partial volume of tissue x.

Note that we do not strictly need the CSF term, since the CSF contribution to the difference signal should be zero. However, the partial volume of CSF is important because it scales the contribution of gray and white matter.

PV correction requires us to estimate both the gray and white matter signal contributions from the difference signal, but that requires us to estimate two unknowns from one measurement, which we cannot do—our system is "underdetermined." We can, however, write this equation for the difference signal in every voxel. If we were to take a group of voxels that were all located close to each other and make the assumption that both the gray and white matter perfusion were the same in all of them, then we would have a set of simultaneous equations. We can ensure that the number of equations (voxels) we use exceeds the number of unknowns (two), and where the number of measurements exceeds the number of unknowns we can get the solution with the least squared error, which then helps reduce the effect of noise on the measurements. This can be written in matrix form as

$$\Delta \mathbf{M} = \mathbf{P}\delta \mathbf{M}$$

where

$\Delta \mathbf{M}$ is the vector of measured difference within a chosen group of n voxels,
$\delta \mathbf{M}$ is the (2 × 1) matrix of unknown gray and white matter difference signal contributions, and
$\mathbf{P}$ is the (n × 2) matrix of PV estimates in each voxel.

This can be solved in matrix form:

$$\delta \mathbf{M} = \mathbf{P}^{\dagger}\Delta \mathbf{M}$$

where $\mathbf{P}^{\dagger}$ is the matrix pseudo-inverse of $\mathbf{P}$.

This solution relies on the matrix $\mathbf{P}$ being well conditioned and will perform poorly if that is not the case. This would happen if all the voxels within the group had very similar PV values, which is unlikely in practice.

In theory, any grouping of voxels can be used in this method. It makes sense to choose neighboring voxels, relying on the fact that the closer in space voxels are the more likely they are to have similar gray matter perfusion. Typically a 2D grid of voxels within an axial plane have been used with sizes varying from 3 × 3 to 11 × 11, largely motivated by the poorer slice resolution of most ASL acquisitions.

This procedure inevitably introduces a degree of spatial smoothing into the final perfusion image that depends upon the size of the kernel employed. This is because, even though we calculate gray matter perfusion in every voxel, each time we do so we assume that the values are similar at neighboring voxels. Unlike most spatial smoothing methods applied to images, such as that considered in Section 3.4, this is not purely a function of the size of the kernel, but also the relative PV values within the voxels. Additionally, no difference in weighting is applied to voxels that are further from the one in the center, nor are voxels weighted based on the consistency with the group or the quality of the data. For example, if the region spanned a discontinuity in the perfusion image, it might be preferable to identify a subset of voxels that were distinctly different to the rest and exclude those from the linear regression to avoid smoothing over the discontinuity. Examples of how the linear regression method performs under simulated conditions are shown in Figure 6.6. An illustration of linear-regression-based correction for PV effects is given in Example Box 6.2.

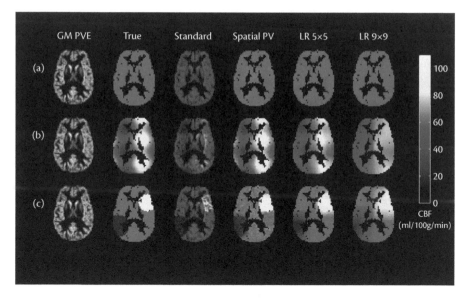

Figure 6.6: A comparison of PV correction methods for ASL applied to simulated data. The original gray matter PV values and gray matter perfusion maps are shown on the left. Various perfusion quantification techniques are shown on the right, including no PV correction (Standard), a spatial prior solution in a Bayesian inference scheme (Spatial PV), and linear regression PV correction (LR) at two different kernel sizes (5 × 5 voxels in-plane or 9 × 9). These results were produced on data that assumed pASL labeling and multi-TI measurements.

Reproduced with permission from Chappell, M. A., Groves, A. R., Macintosh, B. J., Donahue, M. J., Jezzard, P., & Woolrich, M. W., 'Partial volume correction of multiple inversion time arterial spin labeling MRI data', *Magnetic Resonance in Medicine*, Volume 65, Issue 4, pp. 1173–1183, DOI: 10.1002/mrm.22641, Copyright © 2011 Wiley-Liss, Inc.

Example Box 6.2: **Linear-regression-based correction for PV effects**

Figure 6.7 shows the effect of linear-regression-based PV correction, comparing the conventional perfusion image from the single-PLD data from Chapter 1 on the left and the corrected gray matter perfusion image on the right. Notice that the correction tends to increase the perfusion values, and that the gray matter perfusion map is also very smooth by comparison, a combined effect of removing the modulation by the brain structure in the image and also the smoothing caused by the linear regression approach.

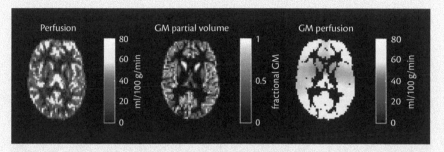

Figure 6.7: Conventional perfusion image from the single-PLD data introduced in Chapter 1 (left), with the image of estimated PVs of gray matter, at the same resolution as the ASL data (center) and the estimated gray matter perfusion (masked by the gray matter PVs thresholded at 10%) using linear regression correction.

On the primer website, you will find the data used in this chapter, along with instructions on how to perform PV correction.

6.2.2 The spatial prior solution

In Section 4.7, we met the idea of spatial priors, which exploited the local spatial homogeneity of the perfusion image to improve the estimates. The linear regression approach already discussed can be seen to be similar. However, the advantages of the spatial prior were that it was applied to the perfusion image not the data and that it was adaptive, such that features and detail present in the perfusion image could be retained. These are all features that are important in the case of PV correction, only now we have two perfusion images to estimate. We can apply spatial priors in the Bayesian-based estimation method on a model that includes both gray and white matter ASL contributions with spatial priors on both gray and white matter perfusion values. The resulting PV-corrected images are then generated based on the use of the spatial information, but it is no longer necessary to specify a kernel size; instead, this is effectively selected automatically and adaptively based on the data. The use of a prior also means that the data plays a role in determining in every voxel which neighbors contribute, and by how much, to the estimated perfusion, further making the process adaptive. The difference in the smoothing that can be achieved on simulated data using this approach compared to linear regression can be seen in Figure 6.6 (although it should be noted that this figure was produced from multi-TI pASL data that provides further ability to separate components, as discussed in Section 6.2.3). An illustration of spatial-prior-based correction for PV effects is given in Example Box 6.3.

Example Box 6.3: Spatial-prior-based correction for PV effects

Figure 6.8 shows the effect of PV correction using spatial priors within a Bayesian inference method for perfusion quantification as introduced in Chapter 4. The gray matter perfusion image is noticeably less smooth than the linear regression solution in Figure 6.7, although the overall pattern is similar, but the maximum gray matter perfusion values are higher.

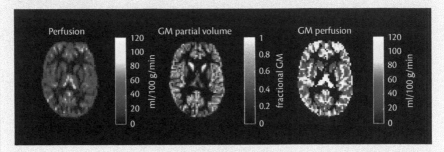

Figure 6.8: Conventional CBF image from the single-PLD data introduced in Chapter 1 (left), with the image of estimated PVs of gray matter, at the same resolution as the ASL data (center) and the estimated gray matter perfusion (masked by the gray matter thresholded at 10%) using PV correction based on spatial priors within a Bayesian inference method. Note the change in color scale compared with previous views of perfusion in this subject.

On the primer website, you will find the data used in this chapter, along with instructions on how to perform PV correction.

6.2.3 Exploiting temporal information

If we have multi-PLD data, we can exploit the extra information provided by the different time points to help improve the separation of gray and white matter components within the kinetic model in the Bayesian inference with spatial priors. As before, both gray and white matter contribute signal to the data, but the kinetics of the two makes their contributions more distinct as a function of time. The differentiating features are the later arrival of blood in white matter along with its shorter T_1. On their own, these features are not sufficient to reliably separate gray and white matter from multi-PLD data; however, they do provide extra sensitivity when coupled with spatial priors. An illustration of spatial-prior-based correction for PV effects on multi-PLD data is given in Example Box 6.4.

Example Box 6.4: Spatial-prior-based correction for PV effects on multi-PLD pcASL

Figure 6.9 shows the effect of PV correction using spatial priors within a Bayesian inference method for perfusion quantification for the multi-PLD pcASL data introduced in Chapter 4. The estimated gray matter perfusion estimate is similar to that derived from the matching single-PLD data in Figure 6.8. The greater sensitivity to ATT in the multi-PLD data improves the ability to separate gray and white matter contributions; thus, it is more reasonable to examine the white matter perfusion map, as shown on the right of Figure 6.9.

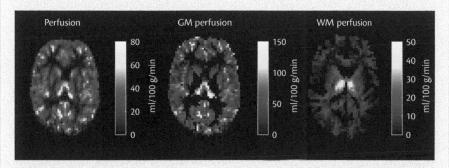

Figure 6.9: The conventional perfusion image (using spatial priors for the perfusion image estimation) from the multi-PLD data introduced in Chapter 4 (left), with estimated gray matter (center) and white matter (right) perfusion images using PV correction based on spatial priors within a Bayesian inference method. As with the single-PLD data, the gray matter perfusion map from the spatial prior method contains more spatial detail than that using linear regression, and there remains some apparent variability in gray matter perfusion across the brain, even accounting for PV effects. As expected, the white matter perfusion is lower than that of gray matter.

On the primer website, you will find the data used in this chapter, along with instructions on how to perform PV correction.

6.3 PV estimation

The predominant approach to obtain PV estimates is to take a high-resolution structural image, segment into tissue types, and then transform into the same space as the ASL data. While there are drawbacks to this approach, it is widely used because high-resolution structural data is often available and automated segmentation is usually successful at these high resolutions. The disadvantage of getting the PV estimate from a structural image is that it has to be transformed to match the ASL data resolution, which involves successful registration between the ASL data and structural image. Doing this registration with a high degree of accuracy can, as discussed in Section 3.3, be challenging. Additionally, the readout used for structural imaging is almost always different from that used for the ASL data, and thus there will be distortions present in one that are not in the other, potentially leading to errors in regions affected by distortion. Once distortion has been corrected for and a good registration has been carried out, it is also important how the PV estimates are transformed to match the ASL data. Specifically, because the PV estimates are quantitative measures of tissue PV, a conventional linear interpolation, as normally used, is not appropriate; see Box 6.4.

Box 6.4: Transforming PV estimates to ASL resolution

An important part of PV correction is the transformation of the PV estimates from high-resolution into ASL space using the (inverse of the) transformation derived from the registration of ASL data to the structural image. Although it is tempting (and easy) to perform this using the normal (tri-)linear interpolation (see the primer in this series "Introduction to Neuroimaging Analysis"), this does not correctly preserve the information about PV effects present in the high-resolution data in this down-sampling process. This is illustrated in Figure 6.10, where two conventional interpolation schemes are being applied to the transformation of data from a high-resolution grid (red dashed lines) to one of lower resolution (black solid lines). In each case, the estimate evaluated is at the location of the black dot: the center of the "voxel" in the low-resolution grid. For both methods, only a subset of the relevant high-resolution "voxels" that fall within the low-resolution "voxel" contribute to the estimate (shaded green).

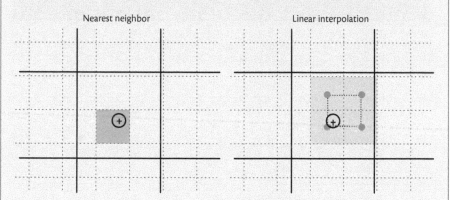

Figure 6.10: Conventional interpolation schemes applied to transformation of high-resolution data (dotted grid) to a lower resolution (solid grid). In both cases, the value assigned to the low-resolution voxel is notionally at the center of the voxel (black circle with cross) and derived only from a subset of the high-resolution voxels contained within its volume (green shading).

A linear interpolation, while perfectly suitable for the transformation of a low-resolution image into one of higher resolution, will not be suitable for the opposite transformation. What we should do is explicitly take the mean over the region in high-resolution space that corresponds to our low-resolution voxel. The low-resolution voxel will inevitably cut through some high-resolution voxels, meaning that we would have to decide whether or not to include these edge voxels in the calculation. A good compromise is to interpolate the high-resolution PV estimate image to an even higher resolution and then perform the integration, thus reducing the overall error in voxels on the boundary of the region. This is illustrated in Figure 6.11: by up-sampling the data, a far larger proportion of the low-resolution "voxel" is informed by voxel values in the (super) high-resolution data.

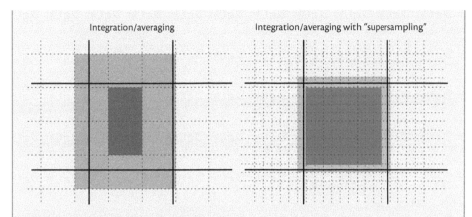

Figure 6.11: Transformation of high-resolution data (dotted grid) to a lower resolution (solid grid) by integration over voxels in the high-resolution images (shaded region: darker shading for high-resolution "voxels" contained entirely within the low-resolution "voxel" and lighter shading for all those that intersect with the low-resolution "voxel"). Greater precision can be achieved by supersampling (blue grid), as shown on the right.

As an alternative to obtaining PV estimates from a structural image, some people have attempted to extract these from their ASL data or from a set of images with the same readout as the ASL data. The main option is to use a series of saturation recovery images, which might form the calibration data (see Box 5.2), to derive a low-resolution T_1-weighted image that can then be segmented. This image will automatically be aligned with the ASL data (except potentially for the need to correct for any head movement), thus avoiding all the issues of registration and transformation. However, the far lower resolution of the data makes accurate PV estimation challenging.

The sensitivity of different correction methods to the PV estimates has not been fully explored, and thus the importance of accurate estimates remains to be established. Currently it is more common to use PV estimates from structural images, largely because these are normally available as part of a study, and the PV estimation itself is relatively routine.

6.4 PV correction and calibration

In principle, PV effects also apply to the image used for calculation of arterial blood magnetization. For calibration using the reference region method, this is not an issue as long as a high threshold has been used to define the reference tissue: which is why CSF and white matter are the most viable choices. For the voxelwise approach, PV effects will lead to different values for the equilibrium magnetization of arterial blood in each voxel based on the proportion of the tissue that would then enter into the final estimated perfusion. Correction could be applied using the methods described in this chapter, but this is less common, primarily because any errors introduced are secondary compared with those in the perfusion image itself. The most likely place for error is around the edge of the brain and near the ventricles, where greater contrast will exist. This leads to a bright rim appearing around the edge of the brain for perfusion images calibrated by the voxelwise approach unless some attempt has been made to correct for this; something that we did in Example Box 5.1.

SUMMARY

- PV effects are an issue for ASL measurements of perfusion because of the relatively large size of the voxels compared with the cortical thickness and because of the marked differences in perfusion between the dominant tissues in the brain.

- Methods exist for PV correction that exploit spatial information to derive a map of "pure" gray matter perfusion (and separately white matter perfusion).

- PV correction relies on good quality partial volume estimates for the tissues. These are normally derived from segmentation of a higher-resolution structural image. Thus, good registration and distortion correction are important to ensure that these estimates can be used with the ASL data.

FURTHER READING

- Asllani, I., Borogovac, A. & Brown, T. R. (2008). Regression algorithm correcting for partial volume effects in arterial spin labeling MRI. *Magnetic Resonance in Medicine*, 60, 1362–1371.
  - *This work introduces the linear regression method for PV correction of ASL images. This work attempts to judge the efficacy of PV correction on in vivo data by introducing an ROI-based quantification of the apparent relationship between gray matter perfusion and gray matter partial volume.*
- Chappell, M. A., Groves, A. R., MacIntosh, B. J., Donahue, M. j., Jezzard, P. & Woolrich, M. W. (2011). Partial volume correction of multiple inversion time arterial spin labeling MRI data. *Magnetic Resonance in Medicine*, 65, 1173–1183.
  - *This work, inspired by the linear regression method, introduces the spatially regularized (Bayesian) solution for PV correction of ASL perfusion images. Comparison of the two methods is made on pASL data with multiple inversion times, used to help improve separation of gray and white matter contributions in the correction process of the spatially regularized method.*

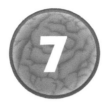

Using ASL to Measure Perfusion Changes in an Individual: Task-Based ASL and Beyond

Thus far, we have been concerned with the estimation of perfusion under steady-state conditions. Effectively, we have been assuming that the perfusion is not varying during the acquisition, normally a period of time of around five minutes. The most typical example is the measurement of perfusion in a resting subject. This chapter considers how we might use ASL to detect changes in perfusion within an individual under different conditions. In the previous chapters, we have outlined the procedure for obtaining a perfusion image using ASL. You could just as easily seek to measure perfusion in the same subject under different physiological states in very much the same way, i.e., perform perfusion imaging under changing experimental conditions with the intent to compare the different conditions or tasks. There is a great deal of flexibility in designing such an ASL experiment; examples of experimental conditions include a continuous visual stimulus (like watching a video) or administering a drug (and watching how perfusion changes as the drug takes effect). In this chapter, we will consider some experimental designs that have been used with ASL. However, there are potentially a much wider range that have yet to be explored that exploit the particular strengths of ASL perfusion measurements.

For all of the cases considered in this chapter, the analysis of perfusion difference, or at least perfusion under different conditions, is performed in an individual subject. If we were then to repeat the experiment on a group (or groups) of subjects, we would consider the analysis that is done within each individual as the "first-level analysis," which extracts measures specific to the individual. A "second-level analysis" to determine whether there are changes in perfusion that are consistent across the group (or between groups, depending on the study) would then be conducted subsequently, details of which are covered in Chapter 8.

7.1 Measuring changes in perfusion

One of the strengths of ASL is that we can repeat the measurement relatively rapidly, i.e., once every few seconds. We know that the brain is dynamic and that neurovascular activity is constantly changing, and thus we may be interested in whether we can infer some of this activity from perfusion measurements. The majority of such functional MRI is based on the blood oxygenation level dependent (BOLD) effect, something that is discussed in more detail in the primer "Introduction to Neuroimaging Analysis". The BOLD fMRI method relies on the relationship between elevated neuronal activity and the associated changes in physiology that meet the increased demand for oxygen needed to sustain it. This effect has been used to study a wide range of behaviors based on participants undertaking a range of tasks or subject to different stimuli. The BOLD effect is itself caused by a combination of changes in perfusion, cerebral blood volume, and rate of oxygen metabolism in the tissue.

We might expect ASL to provide similar information to BOLD, but specifically focused on changes in perfusion alone. Since the BOLD effect relies on changes in blood oxygenation, it tends to have higher sensitivity to the draining veins rather than the specific area of tissue that is showing neuronal activation. ASL, being a measure of delivery to the tissue, might offer better localization. In practice, both are probably sensitive to changes occurring in the capillary bed, and localization differences, if present, are not readily observed with the spatial resolutions currently employed. Additionally, BOLD measurements rely on relative changes in the measured signal between different conditions, such as rest versus stimulation, whereas ASL can provide absolute measures of perfusion. This means that it is more readily possible to interpret the size of perfusion change observed with ASL than it is the relative change in signal observed with BOLD. For example, if a drug causes a larger perfusion change than an alternative, this might be a positive indication of its greater efficacy, whereas we would not be able to say something similar about BOLD changes on their own.

A common BOLD fMRI experiment will alternate the task or stimulation condition every 10–40 s with a rest condition while acquiring images as rapidly as possible. We can take a similar approach with ASL, in which case the analysis steps are similar to BOLD fMRI analysis using the general linear model (GLM); see Section 7.2. This on–off experimental block design is used for BOLD fMRI predominantly because the BOLD signal is not stable over time, even over the relatively short timescale of an fMRI experiment. Drift in the BOLD signal intensity can occur over time owing to changes in the MR scanner, such as those induced by warming of the equipment during the experiment. This means that it is not possible to reliably compare BOLD signal magnitudes from the beginning and end of a single experimental session to look for induced changes—hence the need to interleave periods of rest and task or stimulation over a timescale in which the BOLD signal is approximately stable.

ASL measurements are stable over time for two reasons: first, the ASL perfusion signal is the result of the subtraction of pairs of image, and thus we remove the influence of any drift in the image intensity that causes problems for BOLD fMRI. Second, since we can use ASL to get an absolute measure of perfusion, we remove a range of confounding effects related to scanner setup that might otherwise plague differences in signal intensity seen in different sessions even when carried out on different days. For example, studies have been successfully carried out in which the rest and stimulation conditions were many weeks apart. The stability of ASL-based perfusion measurements means that there are experimental designs where ASL works better than BOLD fMRI; this is especially true for experiments that cannot use the interleaved design needed for BOLD, for example, studies involving the administration of a drug.

The flexibility to perform rest and activation at very different times in ASL studies fulfills a particular scientific role investigating perfusion changes associated with tasks or stimuli that are essentially "one-off", cannot be contained in a short period of time, or cannot be repeated rapidly or even at all. Such studies include pharmacological studies looking at perfusion changes in relation to the introduction of a drug, or physiological studies examining the changes in cerebral perfusion after a bout of aerobic exercise or while performing a learning task.

Where ASL loses out compared with BOLD fMRI is that the time required for an ASL measurement (the repetition time, TR) is longer than BOLD owing to the combination of labeling and waiting for the labeled blood-water to arrive. This reduces the rapidity with which new measurements can be made, something that is made worse by the need to collect label–control pairs. A complete ASL measurement could easily be 7 s (although faster acquisitions can be achieved with pASL or short-label-duration pcASL at the expense of SNR). In comparison, BOLD fMRI measurements can now be made in less than a second. Thus, ASL is not optimal when investigating very fast changes or the small-amplitude changes associated with functional connectivity that are needed for resting-state fMRI analysis (i.e., where no external stimuli or task is required), although resting-state fluctuations have been successfully extracted from ASL data.

The simplest ASL experiments that are designed to measure a change in perfusion are relatively straightforward to analyze. In the situation where ASL data has been separately collected in each condition, a perfusion map (and any other associated image) is calculated for each condition using the methods outlined in previous chapters. An example of analyzing perfusion measurements in a subject when resting and when separately undertaking a task can be found in Example Box 7.1. In the case where the aim is to look at difference across a group, or between groups, multiple perfusion images in each subject, under the different conditions, can be combined within the GLM used for group analysis, as discussed in Chapter 8. However, there are other experimental designs that require specific analysis that we will consider in more detail in the rest of this chapter; an example is tracking changes in perfusion in response to a stimulus for which we do not know ahead of time what the likely time course of perfusion change will be, such as the response to a painful stimulus.

Example Box 7.1: **Perfusion change in response to a task**

Figure 7.1 shows the absolute perfusion changes associated with simultaneous visual stimulation (viewing a flashing checkerboard) and finger tapping in a single subject measured using ASL. In Figure 7.2, the difference between the two conditions has been calculated and overlaid on top of this subject's structural image.

The acquisition for these data was similar to that for the multi-PLD data in Chapter 4, in this case comprising two minutes of ASL measurements when the subject was resting and a further two minutes during the task (96 volumes in each), plus the proton-density-weighted calibration image. The two sets of data were analyzed separately to produce perfusion maps under rest and task/activity, then subtracted to produce the result in Figure 7.2. The perfusion differences between rest and task are relatively noisy, and thus the images here have been masked to exclude changes less than 20 ml/100 g/min, which is an arbitrary choice of threshold for visualization purposes. Localized perfusion increases of up to 50 ml/100 g/min are observed in this case, illustrating that large variations of perfusion in response to stimulus are possible.

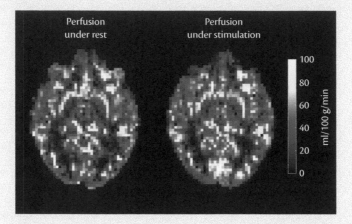

Figure 7.1: Perfusion images under rest and stimulation (during the stimulation condition, the single subject was experiencing visual stimulation and performing a finger-tapping task), measured with multi-PLD pcASL. It is possible to see a region of increased perfusion at the very posterior of the brain, in the occipital region, which would be associated with the visual stimulation.

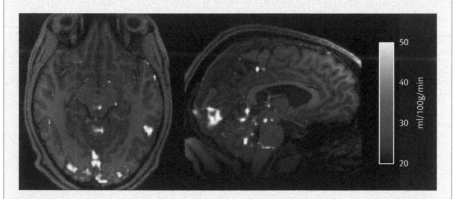

Figure 7.2: Perfusion difference between rest and stimulation (when a single subject was experiencing visual stimulation and performing a finger-tapping task), measured with multi-PLD pcASL. Only changes above 20 ml/100 g/min are shown (to suppress noise for the purposes of visualization). Increases of up to 50 ml/100 g/min under stimulation are observed in this case, and perfusion changes in the occipital cortex are visible, but there is less clear evidence in this single subject of substantial changes in motor regions.

On the primer website, you will find the data from this example, along with instructions on how to compute the perfusion images and the difference image shown here.

The use of ASL to measure perfusion changes associated with a change in physiological status of an individual might require extra care to ensure that it is only perfusion changes that are being reflected in the ASL measurements. While ASL is able to produce an absolute measure of perfusion and thus is relatively robust as a physiological measurement technique, some stimuli can cause non-perfusion changes in the subject that will alter the magnitude of the ASL signal. The main situations about which an experimenter needs to be concerned are the following:

■ Changes in flow speed in the brain-feeding arteries. As we noted in Chapter 2, pcASL labeling efficiency is somewhat sensitive to flow speed in the artery where labeling takes place. A pharmacological intervention, for example, that causes this to alter could result in misleading reports of absolute perfusion changes. Cerebrovascular reactivity studies, which will be discussed in Section 7.5, are a good example of inducing a physiological change that could alter the flow speed in the brain-feeding arteries. Some studies will seek to estimate arterial flow speed to control for this using phase contrast imaging. Note that pASL is relatively insensitive to this effect, although flow speed could change the label duration in acquisitions that do not include QUIPSS II pulses to ensure that the label duration is known.

■ Changes in T_1. It is possible that a pharmacological intervention could alter the T_1 of either blood or tissue and thus lead to apparent differences in perfusion. The influence of changes in T_1 on perfusion quantified from ASL are small in the range of values seen in practice. These differences may be more important when comparing normal with pathological tissue, however.

7.2 Analysis using the GLM

As we have noted, ASL can be used with the typical interleaved design that is usually employed in BOLD fMRI. This includes designs with repeated stimulation/task and rest at regular intervals or designs in which stimulation/task are more irregularly mixed with rest conditions. For simple experiments, it is generally possible to separate the data associated with rest and that associated with stimulation or task, and then compute the separate perfusion images, something that would not generally be feasible with BOLD. In this situation, it is worth avoiding any data collected near to changes in condition (e.g., a change from rest to task), since the perfusion may be varying during this time. However, these changes in condition are something that can be accounted for with a GLM analysis.

More complex designs involving interactions of different conditions benefit from analysis with the GLM, as is common for BOLD fMRI—see the primer "Introduction to Neuroimaging Analysis" and also the online appendix "Short Introduction to the General Linear Model for Neuroimaging." The basic principle of using the GLM to analyze fMRI data is that a linear model is constructed from components that describe the expected time course of the data, for example, a component reflecting the "on/off" activity arising from alternating between stimulus and rest. This linear model is fit to the data, with the amplitude of each component, quantifying the "effect size", being determined from the best fit to the data. The components of the model that capture the signal components expected in the data are often called the "explanatory variables" or "regressors" and are collected together in the "design matrix"; an example design matrix is shown in Figure 7.3. For BOLD data, the task timing details (on/off) are combined with a hemodynamic response function (HRF) that accounts for the assumed physiological link between brain activity and BOLD response. The link between activity and perfusion response is different for perfusion alone, and thus for ASL analysis a different HRF is required, compared with BOLD fMRI.

Since ASL data comprises an alternating series of label and control images, it is still necessary to do subtraction, and this can be done prior to analysis with the GLM or it can be built directly into the GLM as a component of the design matrix. This is done using a specific explanatory variable (EV) that alternates between −1 and +1 every other measurement, with −1 indicating label and +1 indicating control; this is shown as the first column in the design matrix in Figure 7.3. This can then be combined with the experimental design time courses to create specific EVs for the perfusion difference between conditions; this is shown on the right of Figure 7.3. In software, this is often carried out by creating an "interaction" EV between the label–control EV and those describing the experimental design.

In practice, the ASL images themselves will contain some signal related to BOLD that occurs in the static tissue (since ASL images are usually acquired with a readout that includes T_2^* weighting). This BOLD contamination is lost if the ASL data is analyzed after label–control subtraction. However, it is possible to model both ASL and BOLD effects in a single GLM analysis, as shown in Figure 7.3. The advantage of this is that you get all of the following analysis outputs for a single participant:

1. BOLD activation map (statistical test comparing rest and task states).

2. Perfusion image (the mean difference map of the label and control conditions).

3. Perfusion activation map (the difference in the label and control images during the task state compared with the rest state).

The BOLD effect from an ASL acquisition is likely to be weaker than a normal BOLD experiment owing to the use of a shorter TE, which maximizes the ASL signal intensity, but reduces the T_2^* weighting needed for BOLD. This is compounded by the use of background suppression in ASL to suppress artifacts arising from motion and physiological noise (see Section 2.4), which also reduces the BOLD signal. To truly maximize both the ASL and BOLD contributions, it is necessary to design a specific acquisition that acquires both together, such as dual-echo ASL–BOLD, as discussed in Section 7.5.

7.3 Epochs for time-varying responses

There are various experiments that give rise to a time-varying perfusion response that we might like to capture using ASL, a good example being the application of a painful stimulus and the subsequent dynamic changes in perfusion that occur in different regions of the brain. This type of experiment is different to the design we met in Section 7.2 because we do not have a clear expectation of the time course of the perfusion response a priori—this is something that we want to derive from the data. The SNR of ASL data does not provide sufficient precision to reliably extract perfusion at the time of every single measurement (i.e., the result of a single

Single-subject ASL fMRI

| Control tag | BOLD fMRI | ASL fMRI |

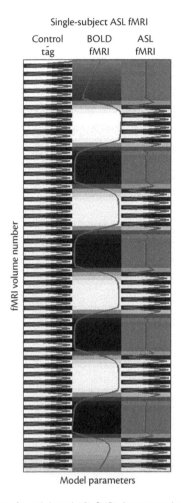

fMRI volume number

Model parameters

Figure 7.3: A first-level analysis of a task-based ASL fMRI dataset can be executed using the GLM. Here the design matrix for such an analysis is shown for a "block design" where the experiment repeatedly alternated between rest and task (five cycles in total). Each row represents a different point in time during the experiments, and hence a volume of fMRI data, with time running from top to bottom of the figure. The experimental design is most easily seen in the middle column. In this figure, the color scale (black–white) and superimposed line (red) in each column indicate the size of the EV, where 0 (black) represents no contribution to the measured signal from the EV at a given point in time. In this example, the three columns in the visualization show the three "explanatory variables" that represent the time courses expected to be seen in the data. The first (left) captures the label–control difference from the ASL label–control pairs and thus represents the contribution from the (resting) cerebral perfusion. The second (center) captures the BOLD effect (which will be seen in the static tissue signal component) arising from the experimental design convolved with the appropriate hemodynamic response function. The third (right) captures the difference in perfusion expected during the task part of the experiment; it has been created by computing the "interaction" between the first column and the task–rest time course (the task–rest timing was combined with the HRF to make the second column for the BOLD effect).

label–control subtraction). A compromise can be found by dividing the data into epochs that contain a number of label–control measurements, as a subset of the full data, from which a perfusion image can be calculated. These epochs can be overlapping and it is even possible to use this strategy with multi-PLD data and thereby extract ATT too. The individual perfusion images obtained by this strategy will still be noisier than a single perfusion image derived from the full data and thus may be harder to interpret. Better SNR is achieved by making the epochs longer, including more individual label–control pairs, but at the expense of temporal resolution, since each resulting perfusion image will correspond to a longer period of measurement time and thus will smooth over more rapid changes. An example of an epoch-based division of resting ASL data is shown in Example Box 7.2. An alternative would be to adopt a GLM type of analysis specifically designed for tasks with an unpredictable time course.

Example Box 7.2: An epoch analysis of single-PLD pcASL

Figure 7.4 shows the single-PLD pcASL data from Chapter 1 once it has been divided up into epochs of 10 measurements and then perfusion-quantified within each epoch. From 30 label–control pairs, five epochs have been generated, each containing 10 pairs, but overlapping the previous epoch by 5 pairs. In this case (of a resting subject), the perfusion looks similar in all epochs, but some increases can be seen in the later epochs compared with the earlier ones.

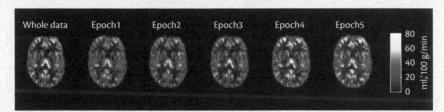

Figure 7.4: The single-PLD pcASL data from Chapter 1 when divided up into epochs of 10 label–control difference images and perfusion-quantified. By visual inspection, we can potentially identify that there are brain regions where the perfusion level has changed over time. We could compare these epochs using statistics, and if we did so, then this would be an example of a "within-subject analysis" (or a first-level analysis).

On the primer website, you will find this dataset, along with instructions on how to quantify perfusion within epochs of the data.

7.4 Dual-echo ASL–BOLD

Dual-echo ASL–BOLD is an fMRI method that deliberately combines ASL and BOLD, attempting to maximize the signal from both perfusion and BOLD effects. We met the idea in Section

7.2 that standard ASL data contains a BOLD component; this occurs as a modulation of the static tissue signal, and thus the BOLD and ASL effects can be separated (the ASL component extracted from subtraction and the BOLD component on the residual static tissue images). However, a compromise has to be made in acquisition regarding the choice of echo time, TE, since a shorter time gives more ASL signal and a longer time increases the BOLD effect (up to an optimal time, beyond which both diminish). A practical alternative is a dual-echo ASL–BOLD acquisition that is achieved by virtue of two echoes, created during the readout phase, and amounting to effectively a twin dataset. A first echo (~10 ms) largely captures the ASL signals, while a later echo (~30 ms) favors BOLD contrast.

The analysis of such data normally proceeds using the GLM, as is the case for BOLD fMRI, since the experimental design is likely to follow the alternating rest/activation pattern suited to BOLD fMRI. The short- and long-echo data are typically analyzed separately for perfusion and BOLD changes, respectively, although combined analyses exist that seek to exploit the small residual BOLD effect seen at the early TE and the ASL component seen at the longer TE. A challenge with dual-echo ASL–BOLD is the tradeoff between good ASL signal and good BOLD signal. In particular, the BOLD signal arises from the static tissue signal that we typically try to suppress in an ASL acquisition using background suppression. It would thus appear that we cannot use background suppression with dual-echo ASL–BOLD acquisitions. In practice, there is some evidence to suggest that the gain from reduction of physiological variability and motion on the ASL, by suppressing subtraction artifacts, outweighs the loss of BOLD signal when some degree of background suppression is used.

7.5 Cerebrovascular reactivity

A cerebrovascular reactivity (CVR) experiment is an example of a specific task-based ASL experiment, but one that is designed to examine a physiological response rather than an underlying functional neurovascular process. The aim is to measure the "reactivity" of the vascular system; essentially, we want to determine what capacity the vasculature has to increase perfusion in response to demand, rather than wanting to find out what increase in perfusion we get in response to a specific functional task, such as attending to a visual stimulation. Hence, a CVR experiment seeks to produce a perfusion change based on a global vascular stimulus, i.e., something that should affect perfusion across the whole of the brain. Like other task-based paradigms that we have considered in this chapter, the CVR experiment consists of a period of rest and another of stimulation, with an ASL perfusion image being acquired in both. CVR is calculated as the difference in perfusion between physiological conditions, and this intensity change is scaled by the rest perfusion to get a percentage difference measure. While we might think of CVR as a way to measure the capacity of the vasculature to respond to demand, it can be both positive (an increase in perfusion in response to stimulation) or negative (decrease in perfusion) depending upon the stimulation used, for example caffeine is known to reduce whole-brain perfusion.

A number of vascular stimulation paradigms can be used for CVR: a classic CVR experiment involves taking a drug called acetazolamide. This agent causes vasodilation, which in turns leads to an increase in perfusion due to a well-established phenomenon called Grubb's law (steady-state flow and volume levels are linked). However, caffeine is also recognized as having a substantial and measureable effect on cerebral perfusion and has been used in CVR studies. Another common CVR experiment involves carbon dioxide (CO_2) gas as a vasodilating agent. Such a CVR experiment is thus based on inducing hypercapnia (the most common CVR approach in MRI studies) or hypocapnia (less common, and a vasoconstriction approach). ASL–CVR with CO_2 gas administration can be used to quantify the change in perfusion per unit change in the partial pressure of CO_2 in the blood by taking a measure of this (normally via measuring the CO_2 in the gases breathed out by the subject). A 5% increase in CO_2 can easily produce a perfusion increase of 50% and beyond in a healthy brain, making it easy to detect a change and thus calculate CVR from ASL perfusion measurements. It is therefore a powerful

Table 7.1 Summary of selected cerebrovascular reactivity values reported from ASL studies (PubMed search criteria: "cerebrovascular reactivity" and "arterial spin" and ("blood flow" or perfusion)).

Paper details	Study details	Baseline CBF (ml/100 g/min)	CBF change (ml/100 g/min)	ASL CVR (% or %/mmHg)	PubMed link
Heijtel et al. (2014)	5% CO_2 gas	51 ± 6.5	13	2.8 ± 1.2	https://www.ncbi.nlm.nih.gov/pubmed/24531046
MacIntosh et al. (2008)	Remifentanyl (drug)	62 ± 12	22	5.7 ± 1.6	https://www.ncbi.nlm.nih.gov/pubmed/18506198
Vidyasagar et al. (2013)	Caffeine	38 ± 5	−7	−2.1 ± 1.8	https://www.ncbi.nlm.nih.gov/pubmed/23486295
Yun et al. (2016)*	Acetazolamide (drug)	39 ± 14	5	−8 ± 4%	https://www.ncbi.nlm.nih.gov/pubmed/26197057
Bokkers et al. (2010)*	Acetazolamide (drug)	45 ± 2	16	36 ± 3%	https://www.ncbi.nlm.nih.gov/pubmed/20574097
Inoue et al. (2014)	Acetazolamide (drug)	49 ± 6	49	44 ± 8%	https://www.ncbi.nlm.nih.gov/pubmed/24371025

* indicates the paper is a patient study.

stimulus for a CVR experiment, although hypercapnia is not always widely appreciated by study participants, since it leads to a feeling of shortness of breath. Some examples of CVR studies and associated summary results are given in Table 7.1.

As noted in Section 7.1, changes in physiology apart from perfusion can give rise to apparent changes in perfusion as measured by ASL. This is particularly relevant to CVR studies where an agent is used to generate a change in perfusion, but where these agents often act by changing properties of the vasculature, e.g., via vasodilation. It is therefore likely that there will be changes in flow speed in the brain-feeding arteries, which in turn will have an impact on the inversion efficiency of a pcASL labeling scheme. For CVR, it may be important to control for this effect using a separate measurement of inversion efficiency or flow speed, but there is currently no agreed standard way to do this. In principle, pASL is less sensitive to this effect if the label duration has been limited using QUIPSS II or an equivalent method, although, if flow speed increases sufficiently, the label may have entered the brain before the QUIPSS II pulses are applied.

SUMMARY

- ASL can be used to detect changes in cerebral perfusion in response to a range of different conditions, including functional brain activity and pharmacological intervention.

- ASL permits a flexible range of experimental designs. The stability of quantitative perfusion measurements provided by ASL means that data from different conditions can be collected at separate times, which can be very widely separated.

- For ASL-based fMRI, the traditional block design of BOLD fMRI is not required, owing to the stability of the ASL perfusion measurement.

- ASL is more suitable than BOLD fMRI for tracking slowly varying changes, e.g., in response to pain. However, it is less well suited, compared with BOLD, for rapid changes that occur over periods of seconds or tens of seconds.

- An epoch-based analysis of ASL data can be used to examine fluctuations and changes in perfusion during the course of an experiment, such as when the response time course cannot be predicted a priori, e.g., a drug infusion.

- ASL, when combined with a suitable pharmacological intervention such as acetazolamide or breathing CO_2, can be used to measure the physiological response known as cerebrovascular reactivity.

FURTHER READING

- Wang, J., Aguirre, G. K., Kimberg, D. Y., Roc, A. C., Li, L. & Detre, J. A. (2003). Arterial spin labeling perfusion fMRI with very low task frequency. *Magnetic Resonance in Medicine*, 49(5),796–802.

- *This paper was one of the first to demonstrate the versatility of task-based functional ASL. It shows that ASL can detect perfusion differences in motor cortex activation over periods of minutes, hours, and even days.*

■ Owen, D. G., Bureau, Y., Thomas, A. W., Prato, F. S. & St. Lawrence, K. S. (2008). Quantification of pain-induced changes in cerebral blood flow by perfusion MRI. *Pain*, 136, 85–96.
  - *This was the first application of single-PLD ASL to image experimental pain in healthy subjects.*

■ Segerdahl, A. R., Xie, J., Paterson, K., Ramirez, J. D., Tracey, I. & Bennett, D. L. H. (2012). Imaging the neural correlates of neuropathic pain and pleasurable relief associated with inherited erythromelalgia in a single subject with quantitative arterial spin labeling. *Pain*, 153, 1122–1127.
  - *This was a multi-PLD pCASL study to image a very rare pain condition associated with a genetic disorder. The multi-PLD method allowed the investigators to interrogate brain function in a single subject.*

■ Segerdahl, A. R., Mezue, M., Okell, T. W., Farrar, J. T. & Tracey, I. (2015). The dorsal posterior insula subserves a fundamental role in human pain. *Nature Neuroscience*, 18, 499–500.
  - *This study employed a multi-PLD pCASL method to quantify dynamic changes in CBF related to a slowly fluctuating tonic heat paradigm that persisted for nearly two hours.*

■ Hodkinson, D. J., Khawaja, N., O'Daly, O., Thacker, M. A., Zelaya, F. O., Wooldridge, C. L., Renton, T. F., Williams, S. C. R. & Howard, M. A. (2015). Cerebral analgesic response to nonsteroidal anti-inflammatory drug ibuprofen: *Pain*, 156, 1301–1310.
  - *This is an example of single-PLD method being used in conjunction with a non-CNS-penetrating drug.*

■ Woolrich, M. W., Chiarelli, P., Gallichan, D., Perthen, J. & Liu, T. T. (2006). Bayesian inference of hemodynamic changes in functional arterial spin labeling data. *Magnetic Resonance in Medicine*, 56(4), 891–906.
  - *This paper seeks to model the combined effects of BOLD and ASL signal differences when using dual-echo ASL–BOLD acquisition.*

■ Ghariq, E., Chappell, M. A., Schmid, S., Teeuwisse, W. M. & van Osch, M. J. P. (2014). Effects of background suppression on the sensitivity of dual-echo arterial spin labeling MRI for BOLD and CBF signal changes. *NeuroImage*, 103, 316–322.
  - *This paper examines the use of dual-echo ASL–BOLD, specifically addressing the tradeoff in ASL and BOLD signal components when background suppression is applied.*

■ Bokkers, R. P., van Osch, M. J., Klijn, C. J., Kappelle, L. J. & Hendrikse, J. (2014). Cerebrovascular reactivity within perfusion territories in patients with an internal carotid artery occlusion. *Journal of Neurology, Neurosurgery and Psychiatry*, 82(9): 1011–1016.
  - *This paper uses the drug acetazolamide to elicit perfusion increases in the brain among healthy adults and patients with occluded arteries. Cerebrovascular reactivity is shown to be impaired in the patient group. Normal reactivity tends to produce a 50% increase in perfusion, while impaired reactivity is roughly half this increase.*

Using ASL to Measure Perfusion in and between Groups of Individuals

Thus far in this primer, we have considered how to obtain measurements of absolute perfusion using ASL in an individual and how to use ASL to detect changes brought about by brain activity or some other form of stimulus. For neuroimaging research studies, these measurements are normally obtained from a set of individuals with the aim of examining perfusion or changes in perfusion within or between different groups. These groups may represent the population at large, or specific subpopulations, such as patients with a particular pathology.

In this chapter, we discuss important things to consider if your aim is to perform a group analysis using ASL data. We will begin by considering the most likely ASL group analysis scenario, which is a single image from each subject of absolute perfusion (i.e., in our conventional units of ml/100 g tissue/min). A fairly natural extension to this is having multiple images from the same subject in different sessions or under different physiological conditions, as in Chapter 7.

The aim of this chapter is not to describe all the details of how a group analysis should be performed. We will assume that you are able to either extract summary measures from your data (e.g., global perfusion or perfusion within a specific brain region) or get all of your perfusion images into the same space (a template or standard space) using registration as discussed in Chapter 3. Once the data is in the required form, group analysis normally proceeds by expressing the relationship between the measurements/images within each group in the form of the general linear model (GLM), with components of the model encoding relationships such as group membership (e.g., patients or controls) or confounds such as age or body mass index. Example Box 8.1 shows such a GLM design from an ASL study. The magnitude of the components in the GLM, which are estimated from fitting the data, capture how much of the differences in the measurements can be ascribed to a specific effect that has been included in the model. For more details on the GLM and how it is used in group studies, you might like to consult the online Primer Appendix "Short Introduction to the General Linear Model for Neuroimaging," and if this area is new to you, we suggest you read that (or another equivalent introduction) before proceeding further.

Example Box 8.1: **Setting up the GLM for ASL group analysis**

We typically use the GLM to capture sources of variation in the data that would explain the differences we see in the perfusion measurements. It is typical to visualize how the GLM is set up, and this is done by plotting the entries in what is called the design matrix. Columns in this design matrix correspond to features in the data that you want to explain or account for. Rows correspond to one participant in one session, which would result in a row for every participant or in multiple rows per participant if we have multiple measurements (e.g., sessions) from each participant (e.g., if you are testing differences pre- and post-treatment in patients). Measurements from each ROI or voxel are treated separately, i.e., the GLM is used separately for each ROI/voxel.

A design matrix for a simple group study is visualized in Figure 8.1. This study comprises two groups (e.g., patients and controls) and thus two columns. For each row, the design matrix in this example takes a value of either 0 or 1 (it represents a categorical variable), indicating whether that individual (measurement) belongs to group 1 or group 2.

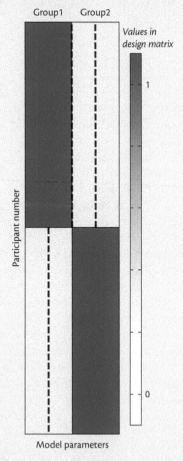

Figure 8.1: Visual representation of a design matrix from a simple study where there are two groups of participants. Note that we are using different colors for this design matrix than in Figure 7.3: here the rows correspond to individuals in the study rather than to points in time during an experiment.

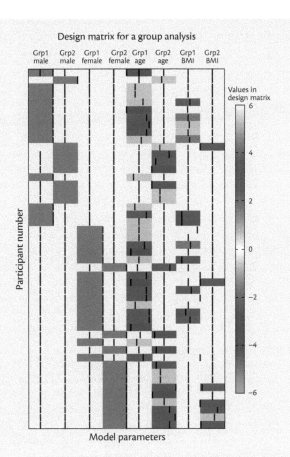

Figure 8.2: This is a more complicated example of a design matrix; here there are eight parameters in the model, represented by the eight columns. This particular model is one that can be used to test for an effect of group, sex, age, and BMI, although there would be other ways to represent the same variable, depending upon the nature of the groups involved and the specific hypotheses being tested (for more information, see the online Primer Appendix "Short Introduction to the General Linear Model for Neuroimaging").

Figure 8.2 shows the design matrix from a more complex study. As before, each row corresponds to a different participant in the study. Columns 1–4 are categorical, and hence 0 or 1. The participant can now belong to one of four groups, since the study seeks to distinguish not only between two types of participant, but also differences due to sex. Thus, this design would allow for statistical testing not only of perfusion differences between patients and controls, but also of whether these were bigger in women than men, etc. Columns 5–8 are continuous measures of age and body mass index (BMI). These are "confounds" that could give rise to perfusion differences between these individuals but that are not directly associated with the hypothesis we are testing, and hence we want to remove any potential effects they have on the data, which is the purpose of including these confounds. Note that columns 5–8 have been scaled and are "demeaned," in the sense that the sum of each column is zero (so that they model variations around the mean value, similar to what is done when correlating variables).

After the GLM has been fit to the data, it is then possible to determine, using statistical tests, whether these effects can be treated as significant. An important feature of any statistical analysis is first stating the null hypothesis. It is easy to overlook the importance of the null hypothesis in the excitement of doing neuroimaging analysis. However, any conclusions you draw from your data are only valid as long as you understand and respect what having a null hypothesis means. The null hypothesis is a specific statement that the investigator makes about their data that will be supported or refuted after performing the analysis of the perfusion data. Typically, the null hypothesis does not capture the effect we are expecting, rather it describes what happens in the case that our hypothesis of interest (also known as the alternative hypothesis) was wrong. For instance, we might hypothesize that a patient group will have lower perfusion in brain regions within the frontal lobe and that this is the effect we want to test using our data. The null hypothesis would then be that there will be no difference between the groups. In this example, we state the direction of perfusion difference and an expectation of which brain region. Both the direction (lower) and location (frontal) in this case are "good guesses" based on accepted knowledge in the literature.

With the null hypothesis defined, we then test to see if the data support the null hypothesis. Two outcomes can occur: (1) we reject the null hypothesis or (2) we fail to reject the null hypothesis. Consider the latter first, where we conclude that our original hypothesis is not supported by the data. This might not be because our original hypothesis was wrong, we might simply not have acquired sufficient data to observe the effect above noise or individual variability. By contrast, if the data does not support the null hypothesis, we "reject" the null hypothesis, this does not mean that our original hypothesis was right, as there might be another explanation to explain the effect we see that we have not accounted for, but it provides support for our hypothesis.

It is possible that we will reject the null hypothesis incorrectly because we happen to have collected a dataset that by chance does not appear to fit the null hypothesis; we would call this a *false positive*. However many times we repeat a measurement, there will always be occasions when, owing to noise or normal random variation, we will get an apparently extreme value. The extent to which this happens is the *false-positive rate*, and is something we need to control for in the analysis. Hence, at the very least, we need to set a threshold probability with which we are prepared to reject the null hypothesis even when by chance it might still be true.

For imaging studies, there is another aspect to false positives than how many times we repeat the acquisition of images. Each image contains many thousands of measurements corresponding to the different voxels in the image. It would be very easy for apparently statistically significant effects to be observed in a subset of voxels simply by chance, given the large number of measurements made. Thus, an important aspect of statistical testing for neuroimaging data in general, and thus no less for ASL data, is correctly controlling for these *multiple comparisons*. There are a number of established methods to control for multiple comparisons in neuroimaging analysis, most of which exploit the assumption that a group of spatially coherent voxels that are all showing the same effect lend support to the effect being significant at that location. Further details of these methods are beyond this primer (see the online Primer Appendix "Short Introduction to the General Linear Model for Neuroimaging"), but are implemented in any software package that allows you to compute group statistics and are very easy to apply.

Knowing something about brain physiology matters when it comes to group analysis of perfusion data. For instance, white matter CBF is significantly lower than gray matter CBF; as we noted in Chapter 6, the ratio is typically assumed to be 1:3, but could be even greater than this. As we have already seen, this gives rise to partial volume effects and explains why perfusion images looks quite a lot like images of gray matter proportion. This knowledge also helps to guide group analysis, since the low SNR in white matter means that it will take more measurements (a combination of longer acquisition and more subjects) to be able to observe a significant effect if there is one to be found when white matter is included. However, analysis that is limited to the gray matter should be more robust, although the resolution of ASL data will mean that the analysis will still include voxels with some partial white matter volume.

8.1 ROI or voxelwise analysis

There are fundamentally two ways to conduct a group analysis: (1) based on regions of interest (ROI) or (2) by considering each voxel independently. Typically, ROIs are chosen when there is literature to suggest that perfusion is altered in a set of brain regions for a given experiment. An example of this would be to test whether the perfusion changes in motor and auditory brain regions as a group of subjects learn to play a musical instrument. Alternatively, performing a voxelwise analysis seeks to identify where in the brain a difference of effect is localized, as well as to determine the spatial extent of the effect. There are advantages and disadvantages of both approaches, as outlined in Table 8.1.

Table 8.1 Comparing the advantages and disadvantages of regions of interest (ROI) and voxelwise group analyses of ASL data.

Group analysis	Advantages	Disadvantages
ROI analysis	■ Implementation: analysis can be performed using statistical software of choice ■ Methodological rigor: ROIs are defined a priori ■ Easy interpretation: average perfusion within the ROI has reduced, increased, or not changed	■ Challenges of identifying ROIs and the possibility of missing an important ROI ■ It is not clear how to include partial volume effects as a covariate
Voxelwise analysis	■ Discovery: each voxel gets due consideration ■ Insight: can identify spatial patterns of altered perfusion ■ Methods: multivariate analysis works well with more measures and more voxels	■ Correcting for the multiple comparisons means an increased risk of false negatives, particularly for voxels with a small effect size

Largely, the choice for an ASL analysis is the same as would be made for any other neuro-imaging study, such as one using BOLD-based fMRI or diffusion tensor imaging. The unique feature of ASL is that, as long as suitable calibration data is acquired, maps or values within the ROIs are quantitative measures of perfusion. This means that it is possible not only to seek statistically significant differences or effects from the GLM analysis, but also to quantify the size of that effect in terms of a meaningful physiological quantity.

8.2 Align your images first

For a meaningful group analysis, each perfusion image must be aligned to a standard coordinate space so that the statistical comparisons are done within equivalent brain regions, i.e., so that the anatomy in the voxels lines up across the group. This is most obvious for a voxelwise analysis, where we need to ensure we are making a comparison within the GLM of the same location in the brain in all the subjects. However, it remains important in many ROI-based studies, since commonly the ROI will be derived from an atlas of brain regions that will be defined in some existing standard or template space.

Alignment requires registration of the data to a template or standard image. More details on registration can be found in the primer "Introduction to Neuroimaging Analysis," but it is likely that you will be registering your low-resolution ASL data to a structural image of the same subject, as discussed in Chapter 3, and separately registering the structural image to the template, since this process is usually most robust. You should always consider what reference brain you are using; it might be reasonable to use a standard anatomical reference image, like the MNI152 standard brain, but how valid that decision is will depend on your participants. For example, the elderly brain is quite different to the young adult brain. You might therefore choose to use a template image that is derived directly from your sample, like a group average, or you could use another established template.

For group analysis, the images are often all transformed to the same resolution as the standard or template image. Since this is normally based on some form of structural image, it will typically be at much higher resolution that the original ASL data. It is often quite practical to use this higher resolution when applying a set of ROIs that have been defined in the standard or template space, since this avoids the need to interpolate the masks that represent each ROI, which can lead to growth or shrinkage of the ROI depending upon how the final mask is generated from the transformed and interpolated result. For voxelwise analysis, more care should be taken when interpreting the group results, since the apparent resolution of the maps of perfusion difference or perfusion effect will be a lot higher than the original resolution of the data. It is common to apply spatial smoothing to transformed perfusion images for voxelwise group analysis, and this can help suppress noise, but also reduces the spatial specificity of any effect found.

8.3 Absolute or normalized perfusion images

Intensity normalization as a final step prior to performing a group analysis is quite a common approach in the literature for a wide variety of neuroimaging methods. Unlike many other methods, ASL offers quantitative measures of absolute perfusion; thus, intensity normalization is not a required step, and in doing so information on absolute difference between groups of effect sizes is lost, although in certain circumstances it may still be advisable—something we will consider in this section.

Intensity normalization is a strategy to ensure that each image has the same global value: which is to say that some value derived from a combination of the voxels, typically the whole brain mean value, is the same (arbitrary) number for all participants. This approach is either necessary or valuable when the global intensity values between participants are different for reasons that cannot be adjusted for or quantified easily. For instance, with SPECT or PET, it may be necessary to sample blood in an artery during the acquisition in order to generate absolute perfusion images. This involves additional setup and is less well tolerated by the patient, so quite often experimenters choose not to do this part. The PET perfusion image then has relative intensity units, which will depend upon the individual, scanner, acquisition parameters, etc., and need to be referenced to a set value for each participant prior to the group analysis. In fact, doing a group analysis on PET perfusion data that does not have intensity-normalized values could produce very odd and unusable findings.

As we have seen, perfusion quantification using ASL does not involve sampling blood or other cumbersome procedures—absolute measurements only require the additional information from a calibration image. By having absolute values of perfusion, we have already controlled for variations due to the scanner, and therefore intensity normalization is not required to correct for such effects.

Despite this, intensity normalization in ASL is still sometimes useful. The main reason to intensity-normalize ASL data is to reduce large variability in global perfusion between participants, due to physiological variability. If the variability in perfusion between individuals is high in a voxel because the global values are vastly different between individuals, then this will impact the sensitivity we have to detect specific differences or effects of interest in the group analysis. Hence normalizing the global intensity should improve voxelwise detection. The tradeoff is that we lose the ability to quantify global differences, because we have essentially made global levels equal for all participants. Thus, if we are examining two groups, for example, patients and controls, it is quite reasonable that the disease process causes a global change in perfusion in the patients, and this is something we might want to detect. However, on the other hand, variability between the individuals might be so high that we cannot detect focal changes in a specific brain region unless we have first corrected for this variability via intensity normalization.

It is up to the experimenter to choose the parameter that will be used for intensity normalization. In most neuroimaging modalities, this would simply be the mean value taken across the whole brain. However, this might not be quite so appropriate for perfusion, since this mean will be affected by the proportion of gray and white matter, and by CSF in each individual (as discussed in Chapter 6). A more common choice is to use mean gray matter perfusion, which is calculated using a gray matter mask. This still requires some care, since the way in which this gray matter mask is generated will have an impact on the value calculated, and it is essentially impossible with current ASL data resolution to create a "pure" gray matter mask. As discussed in Chapter 6, partial volume estimates of gray matter from a structural image should be transformed to the resolution of the ASL data using integration (and not just linear interpolation) and then a threshold of gray matter chosen. Note that although it is tempting to avoid this partial volume problem by defining the mask using images in the higher resolution of a standard or template space, the partial volume effect remains present in the ASL data and will still affect the calculation of the value.

8.4 Parametric versus non-parametric statistics

For the majority of perfusion studies/voxels, common parametric statistics are suitable because the distribution of perfusion values across the sample should conform to the assumptions made by the parametric tests. Increasingly, neuroimaging studies are moving toward non-parametric testing for group analysis, since these tests make fewer strict assumptions about variability in the data. There are several reasons why non-parametric tests are appealing for ASL group analysis and are thus a recommended option.

For the most part, use of parametric testing is reasonable for ASL data. Perfusion values in gray matter tend to range symmetrically about a mean value, typically between 50 and 70 ml/100g/min, and we generally expect the mean perfusion level in gray matter to be 60 ml/100g/min. Variation in the perfusion measured at a voxel will arise from noise and from genuine differences between subjects, and we might reasonably expect this to be normally distributed within a given population. Thus, if you examine the perfusion values, you are more likely to see a nice bell-shaped distribution as your sample size increases. If the histogram has a noticeable skew away from the mean across the group, then that is an indication that you might need to consider a non-parametric test for the group analysis.

It is worth noting that although we might expect variability in perfusion between sessions in the same subject, or between subjects, to be normally distributed, the same might not be true of perfusion changes such as those arising from a stimulus or due to a disease. The reason for this is that, for physiological reasons, perfusion in brain tissue cannot be zero, and perfusion that is substantially lower than normal for any length of time is likely to lead to injury, but there is not such a strict physiological upper bound on perfusion. So it is possible to see an increase in perfusion by 50% in a region of the brain, for example, due to neuronal activity, but it is not generally possible to see a reduction by 50% below baseline levels under normal and healthy conditions. For this reason, a study that involves brain activity might reasonably expect to observed skewed distributions in perfusion effects, and, likewise, the differences between healthy individuals and patients might exhibit skewed distributions.

A very popular non-parametric method is called permutation testing, which is a rigorous way to conduct ASL group analysis. It frees you from assuming that the perfusion values in each and every voxel can be modeled as a normal distribution. This can be important for the reasons already outlined and because, like many low-SNR measurements, ASL data may have features like structured noise that are not accounted for or not known. Example Box 8.2 gives some examples of groups studies using ASL perfusion using both parametric and non-parametric statistical methods.

Example Box 8.2: **Group analysis of task activity changes in perfusion**

In Example Box 7.1, the perfusion changes associated with a combination of visual stimulation and a motor task (bilateral finger tapping) were examined in a single subject. This subject was part of a group of eight individuals who all undertook the same experiment. This can be analyzed either by calculation of the perfusion differences in each subject and then examining the group mean or as a two-group (rest and stimulation) paired test.

Figure 8.3 shows the mean perfusion increase with stimulation across the group in MNI152 standard space; a lower threshold of 5 ml/100 g/min has been applied to this image for visualization. Perfusion increases are observed in the occipital region and motor areas, as might be expected, but note that further statistical testing is required to determine if this change is significant.

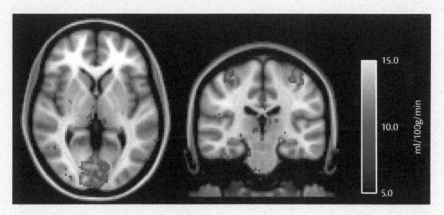

Figure 8.3: Images in MNI152 standard space for changes in absolute perfusion under combined visual stimulation and a finger-tapping task in a group of eight subjects measured using multi-PLD ASL. Perfusion increases in occipital and motor regions are appearing in these images, but the statistical significance of this effect is not reported here.

On the primer website, you will find the data from this study and instructions on how to carry out a group analysis to detect changes in perfusion in response to stimulation, as well as how to test for statistical significance.

8.5 Beyond perfusion

Thus far, we have concentrated on group analysis of perfusion measurements. These could have arisen from either a single- or multi-PLD ASL acquisition. As we have already seen in Chapter 4, using multi-PLD ASL, we also gain information about other hemodynamic parameters, and we might want to analyze these at the group level too. The most probable scenario is that you could examine the ATT maps in a group analysis in addition to the CBF images. This might allow you to detect differences between the groups that are not evident from the perfusion, either because ATT is a more robust parameter for a particular dataset or population, or that differences manifest in changes in ATT rather than changes in perfusion. For example, since ATT is a measure of time of travel for labeled blood-water from the labeling region to the voxel in question, it captures information about the vasculature that supplies the perfusion rather than the perfusion itself. In some patient populations, changes might occur in the vasculature that show up in the ATT measure, but do not substantially alter the perfusion that is maintained by the body so as to permit normal brain functioning.

Group analysis of the ATT images is performed in the same way as for the perfusion images. For consistency, you should use the same group analysis procedure for the ATT data as you do for the perfusion. Keep in mind that you may want to account for "doubling" down on the group analyses and recognize that you are doing two statistical tests on the same data when adjusting for multiple comparisons. You could also look at the ATT and CBF values in each voxel simultaneously in your group analysis, which would be an example of a *multivariate* group analysis, in contrast to two univariate models, one for perfusion and one for ATT, something that is available in some software packages.

8.6 Partial volume effects and group analysis

In Chapter 6, partial volume effects and strategies for correction were discussed. These could potentially be important in the context of group analysis, since they will lead to variations in voxelwise perfusion between individuals that are related to the brain structure and not to perfusion per se. While registration is important when doing group analysis to align the anatomy of the individuals to some common template space, this process does not overcome partial volume effects that arise from the large size of ASL voxels compared with the cortical structure. Thus, even if a perfect alignment could be achieved between individuals, such that all the sulci and gyri were perfectly matched, there could still be a situation, for example, where the measurement in one subject of that tissue happened to coincide with a voxel containing mostly grey matter, but in another it happened to be largely white matter, in which case the reported perfusion values in the template space would be different even if each subject had the same gray matter perfusion at that location. This is illustrated in Figure 8.4, which shows

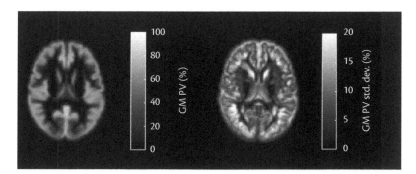

Figure 8.4: An image in MNI152 standard space (2 mm voxel dimensions) of the mean (left) and the standard deviation (right) of gray matter partial volumes across a group of 50 individuals.

variability in gray matter partial volume at every voxel in the MNI125 standard space (2 mm voxel dimension) from a cohort of 50 individuals; see Box 8.1 for more details. Notice that in cortical regions, variability in gray matter partial volume of greater than 15% is possible, and this would correspond to variations of perfusion of the order of 10 ml/100 g/min (if a typical gray matter perfusion of 60 ml/100 g/min is assumed) just arising from differences in the brain structure between individuals.

Box 8.1: Variations in gray matter partial volumes across a group

The images in Figure 8.4 attempt to capture the effect of modulation of perfusion from partial volume of gray matter when group analysis is performed. They were calculated by taking the partial volume estimates of gray matter from T_1-weighted images with a relatively high resolution (1 mm isotropic voxel size), interpolating this to a typical ASL resolution (3 mm isotropic voxel size), and then transforming this low-resolution image into the MNI152 standard space using a nonlinear transformation derived from registering the T_1-weighted image to the MN152 2 mm standard brain. Taking the mean and standard deviation at every voxel across the group produced the images shown. In essence, the standard deviation image shows (at a given voxel in the template space) how variable the composition of tissue in that voxel is between individuals in the group. This has a substantial impact on the measured perfusion, and a substantial component of variability in perfusion across the group is likely to arise from these tissue composition differences, reducing the ability of the study to detect genuine changes or differences of perfusion in the group (or between groups).

The practical implications of this are that the variability of perfusion measurements is likely to be higher than the underlying variability of perfusion in gray matter tissue. Thus, not only will the reported values of perfusion be lower than expected from gray matter, but it will also be more difficult to detect changes or differences in the values. In principle, therefore, partial volume correction prior to group analysis would be expected to improve the ability to detect statistically significant perfusion differences or changes. However, this assumes that further uncertainty is not introduced in the correction process, for example through errors in the partial volume estimates. At present, there are not many examples in the literature where partial volume correction has been applied, and thus the benefits of using it are not yet fully understood. It may well be useful to attempt partial volume correction in any given study, but it remains a good idea to always do a conventional analysis, without correction, as well. One place where partial volume correction may be important is in studies that seek to compare individuals over a wide range of ages or in diseases such as dementia. In both of these cases, changes in brain structure over time (namely, atrophy, which leads to reduced gray matter volumes) will lead to systematic differences in partial volume effects that would manifest as perfusion changes or could mask genuine perfusion changes in a group analysis.

SUMMARY

- Group analysis of ASL data should be the last step after best practices are applied for preprocessing and quantification.

- Group analysis of ASL data shares the same fundamental principles as other neuroimaging group analysis.

- Parametric testing is still widely used for perfusion group studies, but non-parametric testing is increasingly becoming adopted across all areas of neuroimaging.

- It is important to identify and attempt to minimize extraneous sources of CBF variability between participants. One way to do this is through intensity normalization, normally choosing mean gray matter perfusion as the reference, but at the cost of information about absolute perfusion differences.

- ASL data with multiple PLDs can be used to derive other hemodynamic parameters, such as ATT, which can also be used in a group analysis.

- Partial volume effects may lead to greater variability between subjects and thus reduce the ability to detect subtle changes in perfusion. However, correction may also introduce other sources of uncertainty and thus should be evaluated with caution.

FURTHER READING

- Mersov, A. M., Crane, D. E., Chappell, M. A., Black S. E. & MacIntosh, B. J. (2015). Estimating the sample size required to detect an arterial spin labelling magnetic resonance imaging perfusion abnormality in voxel-wise group analyses. *Journal of Neuroscience Methods*, 245, 169–77.
    - *This paper reports on ASL simulation results when using parametric and non-parametric univariate voxelwise statistics. The authors calculate the minimum sample size needed to detect a perfusion deficit as well as to characterize false and true positives.*

- Owen, D. G., Bureau, Y., Thomas, A. W., Prato, F. S. & St. Lawrence, K. S. (2008). Quantification of pain-induced changes in cerebral blood flow by perfusion MRI. *Pain*, 136, 85–96.
    - *This was the first application of single-PLD ASL to image experimental pain in healthy subjects. It was a group study using parametric statistics on perfusion measurements.*

- Segerdahl, A. R., Mezue, M., Okell, T. W., Farrar, J.T. & Tracey, I. (2015). The dorsal posterior insula subserves a fundamental role in human pain. *Nature Neuroscience*, 18, 499–500.
    - *This study employed a multi-PLD pCASL method to quantify dynamic changes in CBF related to a slowly fluctuating tonic heat paradigm that persisted for nearly 2 hours. Using group analysis, it was possible to interrogate which areas of the brain are uniquely capable of tracking fundamental features of the pain experience.*

- Yoshiura, T., Hiwatashi, A., Noguchi, T., Yamashita, K., Ohyagi, Y., Monji, A., Nagao, E., Kamano, H., Togao, O. & Honda, H. (2009). Arterial spin labelling at 3-T MR imaging for detection of individuals with Alzheimer's disease. *European Radiology*, 19(12), 2819–2825.
  - *This paper used pASL QUASAR at 3 T to show CBF differences between controls and adults diagnosed with Alzheimer's disease. In a post hoc test, they make the case that using intensity-normalized CBF images in their group analysis increased the between-group detection sensitivity. As a cautionary note, however, if you analyze your data both ways, you should not then just pick the result you like best, but report on all of them.*

- Binnewijzend, M. A., Kuijer, J. P., Benedictus, M. R., van der Flier, W. M., Wink, A. M., Wattjes, M. P., van Berckel, B. N., Scheltens, P. & Barkhof, F. (2013). Cerebral blood flow measured with 3D pseudocontinuous arterial spin-labeling MR imaging in Alzheimer disease and mild cognitive impairment: a marker for disease severity. *Radiology*, 267(1), 221–230.
  - *This paper compares ASL data between different cognitive groups and reports the findings with and without correction for partial volume effects. Visually, there were noticeable changes to the results after partial volume correction.*

- Nichols, T. E. & Holmes, A. P. (2002). Nonparametric permutation tests for functional neuroimaging: a primer with examples. *Human Brain Mapping*, 15(1), 1–25.
  - *This is a highly cited paper that describes the theory and implementation of voxelwise permutation testing for neuroimaging data. This paper is recommended reading if you are using permutation-based statistics.*

- Bennett, C. M., Wolford, G. L. & Miller, M. B. (2009). The principled control of false positives in neuroimaging. *Social Cognitive and Affective Neuroscience*, 4(4), 417–422.
  - *This paper provides a good overview of the theory of multiple comparison correction. The discussion is on BOLD fMRI data but the same considerations hold for ASL data because both BOLD and ASL rely on similar acquisitions, have comparable spatial resolution and use similar procedures for their group analyses.*

Glossary

3D-gradient and spin echo (3D-GRASE) A 3D imaging technique based on EPI. It does not suffer significantly from signal dropout, but distortions are similar to those in EPI, and through-slice blurring can also be significant, depending on the readout parameters chosen.

Arterial input function (AIF) A mathematical description used in tracer kinetics of the arrival of the tracer in the region of interest as a function of time.

Arterial transit time (ATT) The time it takes the labeled blood-water, the "front" of the bolus for pASL, to travel from the labeling region to the voxel of interest.

> Also known as **arterial arrival time (AAT) and bolus arrival time (BAT).**

ASL White Paper A paper produced in 2015 by the ISMRM Perfusion Study Group and the European Consortium for ASL in Dementia, giving guidelines for a simple, robust implementation of ASL and perfusion quantification for clinical applications.

> Also called the **consensus paper.**

Background suppression The suppression of static tissue signal, commonly used in ASL to reduce physiological noise and motion artifacts.

Calibration (M_0) scan A separate scan in which no ASL labeling or background suppression has been applied. This image is used as a reference to help quantify tissue perfusion in absolute units (e.g., ml/100 g/min).

Cerebral Blood Flow (CBF) Common term for the measured value of perfusion in the brain. Although not strictly a "flow" measurement, it is commonly quoted as ml (blood)/ 100 g (tissue)/ min; it has SI unit of inverse seconds (s^{-1}).

Continuous ASL (cASL) A form of ASL that uses the continuous delivery of radiofrequency to achieve labeling. Most commonly, pcASL is now used in place of cASL.

Control The ASL acquisition in the absence of labeled blood-water. Often used to refer to the image acquired—the control image—in the absence of labeling to be used as a control against which delivery of labeled blood-water can be detected: label–control subtraction.

Echo planar imaging (EPI) A 2D multi-slice MRI technique in which a single slice can be imaged very rapidly (typically ~50 ms). It does, however, typically suffer from signal loss and distortion artifacts due to magnetic field (B_0) inhomogeneity.

Echo time (TE) The time during which the MR signal decays before it is sampled (measured). Typically, a short TE is beneficial for ASL in order to maximize the SNR.

Equilibrium magnetization (M_0) The amount of magnetization at equilibrium in a given tissue or substance. The equilibrium magnetization of arterial blood is an important factor that scales the ASL signal we measure. It can be estimated via the equilibrium magnetization of CSF or tissue, which is easier to measure.

Inflow time The time between the start of labeling and the time of imaging of the voxel of interest. This can be defined the same way for both pcASL and pASL. It has SI unit of seconds.

> It is equal to the inversion time (TI) for pASL or to PLD + LD   for cASL or pcASL.

Inversion time (TI) For pASL, this is the time between the start of labeling and the time of imaging of the voxel of interest. It has SI unit of seconds.

Inversion The "flipping" of the magnetization of arterial water that causes the blood to be "labeled," allowing the detection of perfusion with ASL.

Kinetic model A mathematical description used in tracer kinetics of the concentration of a tracer within a region of interest, as a function of time.

Label duration (LD or τ) The duration of the label as generated by cASL/pcASL labeling, as observed in pASL, or as set by QUIPSS II or Q2TIPS additions to a pASL scheme. It has SI unit of seconds.

Also known as **bolus duration, bolus length, or temporal bolus width.**

Label–control subtraction The process of subtracting two images, one where blood-water has been labeled and one without, to generate an image of perfusion.

Also known as **tag–control subtraction.**

Label/Labeling Blood-water that has been subject to radiofrequency inversion to create a magnetic contrast agent. Also used to refer to the image acquired—the label image after inverted blood-water has been allowed to arrive in the brain.

Also known as **tag/tagging.**

Longitudinal relaxation time (T_1) The "characteristic time" taken for magnetization to recover to its equilibrium state. For ASL, this corresponds to the timescale over which the label decays. Note that after a time T_1, there is still some label left (since the decay is exponential), but if the TI or PLD is more than a few times T_1, there will be little ASL signal left.

Look–Locker An imaging scheme in which multiple images are acquired after each labeling/control period, resulting in multi-delay ASL data. The QUASAR technique uses this method for data acquisition.

Macrovascular signal Signal arising from labeled blood-water within arterial structures that is destined to perfuse tissue at another location.

Magnetization transfer (MT) This process causes a slight reduction in the measured signal, which can occur as part of the labeling procedure, so must be matched in the control condition to avoid control–label differences that are not related to perfusion.

Multi-band A 2D multi-slice technique in which multiple slices are acquired simultaneously, reducing the total time required to image the whole brain.

Also known as **simultaneous multi-slice.**

Partition coefficient (λ) The relative water density in two different tissues, originally defined in positron emission tomography.

Post-labeling delay (PLD) The time between the end of labeling and the time of imaging of the voxel of interest for cASL/pcASL. It has SI unit of seconds.

Pseudo-continuous ASL (pcASL) A version of continuous ASL achieved using a long train of short pulses.

Also known as **pulsed-continuous ASL.**

Pulsed ASL (pASL) A form of ASL that uses a single pulse of radiofrequency applied over a region (e.g., the neck) to label the inflowing blood.

Radiofrequency (RF) The MR signal is produced in the radiofrequency range of the spectrum. Therefore, all coils used to generate or receive the MR signal must be tuned to the radiofrequency range.

Receive coil The piece of hardware that receives the MR signal. It is often designed to fit well to the head to maximize the SNR. Modern receive coils generally have multiple channels, which also boosts SNR, but can introduce a variation in the detected signal across space that must be accounted for when quantifying perfusion or comparing signals in different brain regions.

Also known as **radiofrequency receive coil.**

Relaxation The process of recovery of the magnetization toward its equilibrium state, characterized by longitudinal (T_1) and transverse (T_2) relaxation times.

Repetition time (TR) For ASL acquisition, the time between the acquisition of one image of the whole brain and the next (this includes the time required for the ASL labeling, waiting, and image acquisition).

Residue function A mathematical description used in tracer kinetics to describe what proportion of the tracer is left after its first arrival in the region of interest, as a function of the time since arrival. This is the equivalent of the impulse response function in linear systems theory.

Signal-to-noise ratio (SNR) The ratio of the mean signal (i.e., the true quantity of interest) to the standard deviation of the noise (i.e., random fluctuations that are not of interest). Higher SNR will mean the ASL signal is more easily detectable over the background noise. Note that the value of the SNR will depend on how the signal is defined (i.e., as the signal in the tissue or as the label–control difference signal), where it is measured, and how the noise is calculated.

Spiral A 2D multi-slice technique comparable to EPI. It allows a very short echo time (TE) to be used, but magnetic field inhomogeneity results in blurring rather than distortion. 3D spiral-based methods are also widely used in ASL.

Tag/Tagging Another name for label/labeling.

Transverse relaxation time (T_2 or T_2^*) The "characteristic time" over which the MR signal decays during the imaging process. For spin-echo-based imaging methods, the signal decays with characteristic time T_2. For gradient-echo-based methods, the decay is more rapid, occurring with characteristic time T_2^*, which is shorter than T_2. The echo time (TE) governs how much T_2 or T_2^* decay happens before the signal is acquired.

Index

Tables, figures, and boxes are indicated by an italic *t*, *f*, and *b* following the page number. *vs.* indicates a comparison.